Richard Horton is a physician. He edits the *Lancet,* a weekly medical journal with editorial offices in London and New York. He is an honorary professor at the London School of Hygiene and Tropical Medicine. He is the author of *Second Opinion – Doctors, Diseases and Decisions in Modern Medicine,* also published by Granta Books.

MMR

SCIENCE AND FICTION

Richard Horton

Granta Books
London

Granta Publications, 2/3 Hanover Yard, Noel Road, London N1 8BE

First published in Great Britain by Granta Books 2004

A CIP catalogue record for this book
is available from the British Library.

1 3 5 7 9 10 8 6 4 2

Typeset in AGaramond by M Rules
Printed and bound in Great Britain
by Bookmarque Limited, Croydon, Surrey

For Ingrid and Isobel

CONTENTS

ACKNOWLEDGEMENTS

Thanks are due to many people in many places for helping to shape the events and ideas discussed in this book. First, to my colleagues at the *Lancet* who have provided such strong support and encouragement for much of what appears here. Second, to many of those physicians most closely tied to the controversy surrounding the MMR vaccine. Their availability, often under difficult circumstances, to discuss points of fact, opinion and conjecture is greatly appreciated. Third, to those who formed a wider and more diffuse circle of companionship, sustenance and inspiration. Finally, to those at Granta for offering immediate enthusiasm and wise criticism.

In particular, thank you to Susan Aslan, Virginia Barbour, Robert Beaglehole, John Bignall, Richard Carter, Jessica Clark, Stephanie Clark, Liam Donaldson, Hopelyn Goodwin, Peter Harvey, Brad Hersh, Humphrey Hodgson, Isobel Horton, Astrid James, Tom Jefferson, David King, Sabine Kleinert, Richard Lane, librarians at the Royal Society of Medicine, Ann Löfgren, David McNamee, Robert May, George Miller, Simon Murch, Eldryd Parry, Pia Pini, Drummond Rennie, David Salisbury, Michael Shae, Amali de Silva, Robert Silvers, Sosta, Mike Thomson, Villa Pia (Kevin and Morag), Dominic Vaughan, John Walker-Smith, Lorna Wing, David Wolfe and Ingrid Wolfe.

Quotations that open each chapter are taken from J.G. Nichols' translation of *Thoughts* by Giacomo Leopardi (1798–1837), published by Hesperus Press (2002). Leopardi spent a lifetime reflecting on despair.

'Human society is like fluids. Every particle of a fluid, or tiny drop, pressing strongly on its neighbours above and below and on all sides, and pressing through them on the most distant drops, and being pressed in its turn in the same way, if at some place the resistance and the mutual pushing grow less, not an instant passes before the whole mass of the fluid rushes together towards that place, and the space is occupied by new drops.'

Giacomo Leopardi, *Thoughts*

AUTHOR'S NOTE

This book is an argument that takes its starting point from a precise moment – 28 February 1998. On that day, the *Lancet* published a report that ignited one of the most sectarian debates in modern scientific history. The pleas and propositions that I lay out here represent something of a personal exorcism. A purging of the mind. And not only, I would venture to say, my mind, but also the minds of many of those who have played a part in this singular interruption to the continuity of our understanding about the prevention of human disease. The most controversial part of that notorious 1998 paper was retracted almost exactly six years after its publication, on 6 March 2004. *MMR: Science and Fiction* is my attempt to convert an episode of acute public despair into a declaration of promise and possibility. A reparation, of sorts.

1 August 2004

INTRODUCTION

'Respect is not gained by deference.'

The Vaccine Guide by Randall Neustaedter looks innocuous enough. It is a book with a sober academic cover that can be found in most bookstores. I bought my copy in June 2004, at a café close to University College London. But as soon as the reader turns the cover, they will enter a world of striking half-truths, gross errors of omission and astonishing manipulations of fact. On the first page, you will read this: 'The vaccination campaign has traded infectious diseases of childhood for chronic autoimmune diseases that afflict both children and adults.' One of those gratefully acknowledged by Neustaedter is a doctor called Andrew Wakefield.

Neustaedter asserts that vaccines are 'dangerous', that the 'devastating disease' they cause is 'shocking and scandalous', and that these allegedly terrible adverse reactions are 'constantly suppressed' by the medical establishment. In the chapter devoted to the measles, mumps and rubella (MMR) vaccine, he writes that 'the vaccine is associated with serious adverse reactions including permanent nervous system damage and autism'. He recommends 'alternative healing systems' to treat measles. Elsewhere, Neustaedter comments that 'it should come as no surprise that measles vaccine could also cause an insult to the brain resulting in autism'.

MMR: Science and Fiction aims to set the record straight about the history, safety, and effectiveness of the MMR vaccine. But I also hope to do far more than this. I want to examine the way in which the sometimes vicious personal debate about this vaccine has evolved and what that debate tells us about the place of science in society today. I want to describe the current commercial influences in medical research and how they are scarring vital academic values of independence and impartiality. I want to sketch our present knowledge about autism and what we must do to understand this perplexing condition far better than we do now. I want to take a global look at the huge burden of measles among children in developing world countries and the likelihood that we might one day eradicate measles from the planet. And finally, I want to tease out the often aberrant relationships between science, government, the media and the public. I want to discover just what is the proper place of science in society. In sum, I try to answer this question: what are the prospects for creating a culture in which scientific disputes can proceed openly, responsibly and in proportion to the perceived threat? This is a question that we will have to answer if our society is not to regress into a primitive era of witchcraft and absurdity.

I turned to Andrew Wakefield and remarked, more as a way to break the silence than as a comment in need of a reply, 'It seems like this whole affair is coming to a head.'

It was a baleful understatement, one that not only failed to match the occasion – the imminent implosion of work that had divided parents from their doctors, and even doctors from their colleagues – but also proved premature in its suggestion that the events of the previous six years were soon to be concluded. Perfectly aware of these realities, Wakefield looked past me, expressionless.

We were sitting next to each other in the London offices of the *Lancet* on the afternoon of 18 February 2004. Around a large circular table we had been joined by Professor John Walker-Smith and Dr Simon Murch. Dr Peter Harvey, a neurologist, arrived a little later. They, together with Dr Wakefield, were the senior authors of the 1998 *Lancet* paper that had triggered a cascade of bizarre and catastrophic events,[1] all of which conspired to undermine public confidence in the MMR vaccine. A group of the journal's editors, including myself, had just sat through a gripping five-hour presentation of evidence against Wakefield, his colleagues and the Royal Free Hospital by Brian Deer, a freelance journalist working for the *Sunday Times*. The tension in that earlier meeting had been heightened by the shadowy presence of Dr Evan Harris, a Liberal-Democrat Member of Parliament.

The allegations made by Deer, as I saw them, were devastating. He claimed that a team of doctors led by Wakefield had conducted invasive investigations on children, including lumbar punctures, in which a steel needle is inserted through the child's back between two vertebrae to extract a sample of the fluid that bathes the spinal cord and brain, without the approval of the hospital's ethics committee. Worse still, Deer alleged that these investigations had been completed under the fabricated cover of ethics committee approval for an entirely different study on different children – a charge of deliberate deception against the Royal Free team.

He made the further allegation that the children described in the *Lancet* paper had been invited to take part in the study based on family and medical reports of a temporal association between their child's illness – a previously unreported combination of autism and bowel disease – and the MMR vaccine. If this claim were true, it would have meant that the selection of children who took part in the investigation had been badly biased, leading to an entirely erroneous interpretation that the MMR vaccine might have been the common trigger for the children's illness.

Deer also provided us with evidence suggesting that Wakefield was conducting two quite separate studies at the time of the publication of his 1998 article. One study included the work that we published in the *Lancet*. The other investigation was a Legal Aid Board funded pilot project, agreed between the Board and Wakefield in 1996, which aimed to find evidence to support multiparty litigation against vaccine manufacturers. Deer claimed that Wakefield had been funded by the Legal Aid Board to do this second piece of work, leaving a clear danger that it would be perceived as a conflict of interest for someone who was supposed to be conducting independent investigations as part of a National Health Service and university team of scientists and physicians. Indeed, it was alleged that children in the Legal Aid Board funded project were the same as those described in the *Lancet* paper, a fact that, if true, had not been disclosed to editors of the journal as it should have been.

Wakefield, Walker-Smith and Murch strenuously denied that their work had bypassed ethics committee approval. They explained how a simple misreading of the available documents had led Deer and Harris to misunderstand the circumstances of their investigations. They had indeed had ethics committee approval for the study (see Appendix). They argued that the children had been referred to the Royal Free consecutively – that is, one after the other. They had not been 'cherry-picked' by Wakefield to fit a predetermined theory connecting the MMR vaccine with autism. All of the authors of the 1998 *Lancet* paper rebutted these allegations.

It was true, however, that the referral of some of these children had been unusual. They had not simply turned up at the Royal Free by chance. Some of the parents knew about Wakefield's interests and his prior view that measles was somehow linked to bowel disease. So, although the children reported in the *Lancet* paper had not been deliberately selected based on their parents' belief that the MMR vaccine was linked to their illness, some of the families had actively sought out Wakefield, rendering their child's selection far from random. These complex but important details had been omitted from the original *Lancet* report.

There the consensus ended. Wakefield admitted that he had been commissioned by the Legal Aid Board to conduct a pilot study on behalf of parents of allegedly MMR-vaccine-damaged children. Some of his colleagues claimed that he had not disclosed this fact to them. Simon Murch and John Walker-Smith were visibly shocked by his revelation. Wakefield agreed that some of the children – four or maybe five – described in the *Lancet* paper were also part of the litigation-driven research. And he accepted that he had taken money from the Legal Aid Board – although not the £55,000 alleged by Brian Deer and certainly not for personal gain. A figure of £25,000 was closer to the true sum, he said, and this had passed immediately to the Royal Free to help pay the salary of an assistant who would subsequently complete work on tissue samples to identify (or not) measles virus.

Wakefield maintained that such strange circumstances did not amount to a conflict of interest. He would, he said, eventually declare this funding when the results of the work for which that money had been used were finally reported. I disagreed with him. The issue, to my mind, was whether a perception of a conflict of interest existed. A conflict of interest occurs when an individual's private interests differ from his professional obligations to his patients, his colleagues or his hospital. A conflict of interest is created by a situation, not by a specific action. Such a situation can be dangerous – and must be disclosed in order to be dealt with openly – because a personal interest, often but not exclusively financial (in Wakefield's case it was financial for research funding *and* intellectual), may compromise or present the appearance of compromising an individual's professional independence. Clearly, the perception of a compromise existed here. Wakefield's dual commitment – to the Legal Aid Board and to the Royal Free Hospital – posed dangers that he should have seen and disclosed. He did not.

On the basis of this new evidence, we concluded that had we known in 1998 what we knew now in 2004, 'this information would have been material to our decision-making about the paper's suitability, credibility, and validity for publication'. After we released the results of our investigation and determination, together with statements from Walker-Smith, Murch, Wakefield and the Royal Free Hospital, two days later on Friday, 20 February, I went further.

When asked directly by journalists whether I would have published the 1998 Wakefield paper if I had known then about the perceived conflict of interest, I felt that I had to say more than the carefully worded statement that we had released. It was as if a coil of suppressed frustration was unwinding within me, having been pressed into a position of extraordinary tension during the preceding six years. On the evening of 20 February, I said on BBC television news: 'If we knew then what we know now we certainly would not have published the part of the paper that related to MMR, although I do believe there was and remains validity to the connection between bowel disease and autism.' In other interviews I said: 'There were fatal conflicts of interest in this paper . . . in my judgement it would have been rejected . . . As the father of a three-year-old who has had MMR, I regret hugely the adverse impact this paper has had.' I called Wakefield's work on the link between the

MMR vaccine and autism 'fatally flawed'. The headline in the next day's (21 February) newspapers reflected this more aggressive line. 'Medical journal raps MMR report doctor,' said the *Daily Express*. '*Lancet* in attack on MMR doc,' proclaimed the *Daily Mirror*. 'MMR doctor criticized,' announced *The Times*. '*Lancet* MMR report invalid, says editor,' reported the *Daily Mail*.

A whirlwind of innuendo ensued, which caught all of us in its wake. Evan Harris, the MP who had mysteriously joined Brian Deer at the *Lancet*'s offices, called for an independent inquiry into Wakefield's research. Put on the backfoot by the sudden escalation in media interest and by Harris's calls for a public inquiry, Britain's Health Secretary, John Reid, urged the General Medical Council (GMC, the body that regulates doctors) to investigate Wakefield 'as a matter of urgency'. Even Prime Minister Tony Blair jumped into the debate, saying, 'There is no evidence to support this link between MMR and autism.' The story was by now political, not medical – and unhelpfully so for such an incendiary matter that demanded cool judgement if further public confusion was to be limited.

Indeed, the GMC seemed nonplussed by Reid's intervention. The best their spokeswoman could say was: 'We are concerned by these allegations and will be looking at what action, if any, may be necessary.' In truth, they had not a clue where to begin. At a dinner I attended on 23 February, one medical regulator and I discussed the Wakefield case. He seemed unsure of how the Council could play a useful part in resolving the confusion. As we talked over coffee while the other dinner guests were departing, he scribbled down some possible lines of investigation and passed me his card, suggesting that I contact him directly if anything else sprang to mind. He seemed keen to pursue Wakefield, especially given the ministerial interest. Here was professionally led regulation of doctors in action – notes exchanged over liqueurs in a beautifully wood-panelled room of one of medicine's most venerable institutions.

Journalists now began to personalize as well as to politicize the storm. Wakefield was described as a 'pariah', a 'maverick' and 'a thorn in the side of the public health establishment'. I was labelled an unpredictable 'firebrand' whose 'style of campaigning is not appropriate for the custodian of a great scientific institution, such as the *Lancet*'. I was 'vulnerable'. The pseudonymous columnist Theodore Dalrymple invited readers to 'enjoy the squirming of the *Lancet* while it lasts'. Brian Deer wrote in the *Sunday Times* that 'medical insiders now wonder if he [that is, Horton] can survive the scandal that has damaged the *Lancet*'. (Meanwhile, he was described as 'one of Britain's top investigative journalists'.)

The blistering criticism of Wakefield which our collective announcement had initiated led some parents of children suffering from autism to accuse doctors and the government of a witch-hunt. 'There are sick children,' they said. 'Thanks to Dr Wakefield, they are being treated.'

Liam Donaldson, the Chief Medical Officer, proceeded to wade into a now wholly confused debate by accusing Wakefield of doing 'poor science'. One could see parts of the medical establishment gloating over Wakefield's discomfort. Unfortunately, Donaldson failed to distinguish between the two parts of the 1998 *Lancet* report – first, the more tenuous, and indeed now discredited, link between the MMR vaccine and an autism–bowel syndrome, and second, the new syndrome itself. Donaldson clearly blamed the *Lancet* for causing the entire episode. He said: 'If the paper had never been published, then we wouldn't have had the controversy, we wouldn't have had the seed of doubt sown in parents' minds which has caused a completely false loss of confidence in a vaccine that has saved millions of children's lives around the world.'

A media backlash soon started in the face of these attacks on Wakefield. Writing in the *Daily Express*, Jacqui Jackson, a writer on autism, advised parents: 'MMR: do not take the risk.' Melanie Phillips in the *Daily Mail* accused us all of smearing Wakefield. She commented: 'Although the vast majority of children clearly have no adverse reaction whatever from the MMR jab, the number of families with a very different story to tell indicates that, for a small proportion of children, something worrying may be happening.'

The Autism Research Campaign for Health called for a public inquiry to investigate the safety of the vaccine. Isabella Thomas, one of the parents who first consulted Wakefield in 1996 about her son's deteriorating condition, told London's *Evening Standard*:

> He [Wakefield] was the first doctor who really listened to us. He has been prepared to sacrifice his job and his reputation for justice – his life and that of his family's is now in turmoil. The establishment is trying to vilify the one person who truly believes us – and whose research, no matter who paid for it, revealed a deeply worrying phenomenon . . . this man was my saviour – he wanted to help me whereas others just saw me as the mother of a damaged child, and an 'inconvenience'. Some health professionals said that, as a mother of two sons with behavioural problems, I couldn't control them. It had even been suggested that my husband Ian and I were bad parents.

The *Daily Mail* supported this view. The newspaper called the debate about the validity of Wakefield's original report a 'betrayal of these tragic parents'. They continued to demand that Tony Blair disclose whether his son Leo had received the MMR jab. It was widely suspected, based on little more than rumour and gossip, that Leo had received single vaccines for measles, mumps and rubella separately, perhaps while overseas. Stephen Glover, the *Daily Mail*'s acerbic columnist, called us all 'Assassins'.

More thoughtful writers invited all parties to consider these events with a little more detachment.[2] For example, Lewis Wolpert, a professor of anatomy and developmental biology at University College London and a frequent commentator on the public's understanding of science, asked the *Lancet* to 'consider the consequences and its responsibility carefully'. Indeed, that was just what we were doing.

For if I was now claiming that the interpretation in the 1998 *Lancet* paper concerning the MMR vaccine and autism was entirely flawed – and I was – how could that part of the paper remain on the public record? I discussed the logic of the events as they were unfolding with Simon Murch, one of the original Royal Free team and a respected paediatric gastroenterologist. We agreed that a retraction was needed. But not a retraction of the whole paper. In the world of science, a retraction is the most serious sanction that can befall the work of any scientist. Typically, a retraction is required when there is proven evidence of fraud.

On this occasion, we had discovered an error of judgement, an important error of judgement to be sure: a failure to disclose a perceived conflict of interest that would have almost certainly altered peer reviewers' and editors' views about a preliminary and controversial finding. Did this behaviour amount to scientific misconduct? It was hard to tell. But certainly it invalidated Wakefield's central claim – namely, that the link between the MMR vaccine and autism was a serious independently arrived-at scientific hypothesis that needed to be investigated urgently.

We needed a partial retraction, erasing, as far as one reasonably could, the interpretation concerning the vaccine and autism. None of the factual material described in the 1998 paper was in doubt. Twelve children did exist. Their clinical case histories were not disputed. The findings on physical examination of the children remained unquestioned. The hypothesis that formed the principal conclusion of the paper – that a new syndrome of bowel disease and an autistic-like behavioural disorder had been discovered – was intact, although it still remained a subject of continuing investigation. But the credibility of the interpretation based on these facts had now been totally undermined.

Yet retractions are uncommon. How should we proceed? There is little available guidance for editors. One set of guidelines is published by the International Committee of Medical Journal Editors. It advises that editors should pursue retraction if fraud is detected. The UK's Committee on Publication Ethics, an informal grouping of British and continental European editors, simply advises that 'whenever it is recognized that a significant inaccuracy, misleading statement, or distorted report has been published, it must be corrected promptly and with due prominence'.

There had been examples of partial retractions in the past. A fragment of the total data described in a research paper or a specific illustration or figure, for example. I found the precedent we were searching for in *Science*, a prominent US journal published by the American Association for the Advancement of Science. In January 2004 its editors had published a 'retraction of an interpretation' by a leading group of HIV–AIDS investigators.[3] The premise for the retraction was that, while the facts in their report were unchallenged, the authors' interpretation of those facts was wrong. Such a major error, once discovered, had to be withdrawn. An identical situation faced us now.

Simon Murch managed to convince ten of the original thirteen authors to sign up to this partial retraction. A draft was agreed and submitted to us. Wakefield and Peter Harvey, the neurologist who examined the children in the original study, could not be persuaded to sign, despite, in the case of Wakefield, a personal entreaty – an 'olive branch', I called it – from me. After protracted negotiation, the draft statement was considered too inflammatory. It seemed to lay particular blame on Wakefield for advocating single vaccines in place of the triple MMR vaccine at the press conference called by the Royal Free Hospital to launch the *Lancet* paper. Since it had just been reported in the press that Wakefield had instructed his lawyers to pursue the *Lancet* for an apology,[4] and given that I had gone beyond our originally agreed statements by calling the MMR part of his theory 'fatally flawed', some of those taking part in agreeing the statement of partial retraction were anxious that the statement should be neutral in tone.

We wanted to run the retraction in our 6 March 2004 issue. We were due to go to press at 4 p.m. on 2 March. By lunchtime we still had no finally agreed retraction statement. I called Humphrey Hodgson, the vice-dean of the medical school. He put the matter bluntly: 'What do you need?' he asked. A clear statement of withdrawal from the MMR claim, I said, with the word retraction in the title. 'OK,' he replied. An hour or so later we had the statement we needed.

Ten of the authors wrote: 'We wish to make it clear that in this paper no causal link was established between MMR vaccine and autism as the data were insufficient. However, the possibility of such a link was raised and consequent events have had major implications for public health. In view of this, we consider now is the appropriate time that we should together formally retract the interpretation placed upon these findings in the paper, according to precedent.' Several weeks later, Wakefield, Harvey and John Linnell replied.[5] They argued that Wakefield had not attempted to conceal his work for the Legal Aid Board, that the 1998 *Lancet* article 'was not a scientific paper but a clinical report', and that 'No Legal Aid money was used in the preparation of the 1998 paper'. Concerning the statement that Wakefield made at the Royal Free Hospital's press conference about dividing the MMR vaccine, they wrote: 'We regret the furore and polarization of opinion that ensued from that press briefing for which AJW [Wakefield] bears some responsibility.' All parties were now at last displaying contrition for the events of the previous six years.

Despite my strong misgivings about Andrew Wakefield's judgement during this whole episode, there was something deeply unpleasant about how his public humiliation had unfolded. During the preceding few weeks, one protagonist in the affair had said openly and publicly that his intention was to 'rub out' Wakefield. A senior doctor who had played a part in shaping the debate around MMR sat in a North London bar with a glass of red wine in front of him boasting that he was 'drinking the blood of Andrew Wakefield'.

The intensity of feeling that Wakefield provoked in some of his opponents was unbelievably extreme. And, in the aftermath of the David Kelly affair, in which a British scientist and respected civil servant committed suicide after being caught up in a media blitz following a few incautious remarks to a BBC journalist, only those of a very robust constitution would have been able to stand up to the continued pressure of critics who wished to destroy his reputation. Wakefield's tribulations seemed insufficient for some. Whatever one's views about his wisdom as a doctor and scientist, this kind of malicious reaction somehow seemed equally bad – perhaps even worse.

As I try to show in this book, the Wakefield affair reveals a society undone and unable to come to terms with dissent, uncertainty, the meaning of evidence, the inescapable human need for trust, and our wider global responsibilities. Contrary to the way in which Wakefield's trials have been portrayed, the collapse of the evidence surrounding the MMR vaccine theory of autism is not a triumph of reason over passion. Instead, it illustrates a deep and more general crisis of rationality, an inability to resolve disputes fairly and reasonably in a society whose bonds of altruism, respect and decorous exchange have loosened to a quasi-medieval degree – a crisis that, if left unchecked, will end inevitably in violence and anarchy.

CHAPTER 1

Is the MMR Vaccine Safe?

'There is nothing in the world so false and so absurd that it is not believed to be true by very sensible people, whenever their minds cannot find any way of coming to terms with the opposite and being at peace with it.'

Although measles was recognized as a human disease as far back as the seventh century, it was the Persian physician Rhazes who first gave it a name – 'hasbah', which means 'eruption' in Arabic. He made the important diagnostic distinction between hasbah and smallpox, concluding, incredibly to modern eyes, that smallpox was the rather less dreadful disease. The word 'measles' stems from a long list of etymological corruptions, probably originating from *miser*, the Latin for miserable – a perfectly accurate description of a condition that renders one prostrate with a severe fever, a sore throat and eyes, an irritating and persistent cough, a rash, a runny nose and a general feeling of fatigue, collapse and awfulness.

Thomas Sydenham, the great seventeenth-century English explorer of human fevers, was the first to describe the clinical characteristics of measles, which he believed must be an infectious disease. This belief was finally converted into fact by the ingenious and bold experiments of a Scottish physician, Francis Home. In 1757, he took blood from a patient with measles who had both a fever and the characteristic rash of the condition. He inoculated this person's blood into twelve otherwise healthy children, ten of whom proceeded to develop symptoms and signs typical of measles.[1]

The conclusions of these challenging – and certainly unethical by today's standards – experiments were confirmed by Peter Panum, a Danish doctor who studied a measles epidemic on the Faroe Islands in 1846.[2] He found not only that measles was contagious, but also that infection conferred lifelong immunity. Eventually, over a century later in 1954, the measles virus was tracked down, cornered and isolated by John Enders and Thomas Peebles.[3] This was the discovery that heralded the development of a vaccine.

Why was a vaccine important? Measles is a highly contagious disease, spreading through the air via droplets of fluid from the throat and nose of those affected. It commonly infects children, and caused, at its peak, as many as 500,000 reported cases of the disease annually in the US. So common was measles infection that it was once viewed as a normal part of growing up. Although death from uncomplicated measles is extremely rare in the western world, the condition is unpleasant and carries the risk of several, occasionally fatal, long-term complications.

Measles has three clearly separate phases. First, there is an incubation period – the interval between exposure to the virus and first symptoms – of ten to fourteen days. The second (or prodromal) stage is signalled by the brewing infection boiling up into a nasty stew of fever and symptoms not unlike a severe cold. This phase lasts two to four days. Finally a rash arrives, usually preceded by Koplik spots – whitish-grey flecks on a red base, which are characteristic of measles and appear on the inside of the mouth. The skin rash begins on the face and moves steadily down the body, affecting the palms and soles and continuing for about six days. The entire experience of illness lasts up to ten days.

Complications depend on where in the world one lives and the age at which measles is contracted. In developing countries, measles can kill as many as one in ten of those it infects. The virus causes severe diarrhoea and inflammation of the mouth which, against a background of malnutrition, can be devastating. (I discuss the entirely preventable tragedy of measles in the developing world in Chapter 5.)

In more industrialized nations, complications include ear infections (occurring in 7–9 per cent of cases), pneumonia (1–6 per cent), diarrhoea (6 per cent), and death (0.1–1 case per 1,000 cases of measles infection). The commonest cause of death from measles is pneumonia. Two further complications, although rare, are extremely debilitating. Both involve the measles virus penetrating the brain. Measles encephalitis affects one in 1,000 to one in 2,000 of those who contract the infection. It leaves many of those who survive permanently brain-damaged. Subacute sclerosing panencephalitis (SSPE) is even rarer, affecting one in 100,000 of those infected. Mental and physical decline usually begin about seven years after the primary measles infection, which in half of all cases of SSPE occurs before two years of age. Personality changes, seizures, disability, coma and eventually death ensue.

These complications might seem rare in percentage terms. So what do they add up to? Let us go back to that figure of 500,000 cases of measles each year in the US. In truth, that number was a wild under-estimate. Measles is so contagious that all children became infected at some stage in their early lives. At such a phenomenal attack rate in the pre-vaccine era, measles caused 150,000 respiratory complications, 100,000 ear infections,

48,000 hospitalizations, 7,000 seizures, 4,000 cases of encephalitis (as many as 1,000 of whom were left permanently disabled) and 500 deaths. A vaccine was a vital tool to control this annual epidemic. In the UK, the absolute burden of measles – and mumps and rubella – was more modest, but still substantial and proportionately identical. Measles caused around 850 deaths in England and Wales in the decade before a vaccine was introduced. Rubella causes low birthweight, eye and heart damage, deafness and neurological disabilities and diabetes mellitus. Mumps is a painful condition producing inflammation and tenderness of the salivary glands, testes, or ovaries. Meningitis occurs in half of all cases of mumps. Persisting deafness is a further rare complication.

A live measles vaccine was first licensed for use in the US in 1963. Since then, the incidence of measles has fallen by 99 per cent. There were problems with some of these original vaccines. A killed measles vaccine was licensed at the same time as the live vaccine, but this product had to be withdrawn in 1967 because it allowed an atypical presentation of measles to occur in vaccinated children. The first live vaccine was based on a strain of the virus called Edmonston B, named after the person from whom the virus was isolated. But this vaccine caused unacceptably high rates of fever and rash. More attenuated and therefore safer vaccines had to be developed.

A combination of measles, mumps and rubella (MMR) vaccines was first approved in the US in 1971. It was introduced into the UK in 1988, replacing the single measles vaccine for twelve- to eighteen-month-olds and a rubella vaccine that was given to schoolgirls and adult women. The MMR vaccine led to a rapid decline in remaining measles and rubella infections. The incidence of mumps also fell dramatically. Currently (in 2004), two types of MMR vaccine are available in the UK: MMR II (made by Merck and marketed by

Aventis Pasteur) and Priorix (made by GlaxoSmithKline). The goal of public health authorities is that every child should receive two doses of an MMR vaccine by the time he or she enters primary school.[4]

A first dose of MMR vaccine is given at twelve to fifteen months. A booster dose is given at three to five years, before starting school. A feeling of fatigue, together with a fever or a rash, may occur about a week after vaccination. These symptoms should last no more than a few days. In rare cases, the formation of a particular type of blood cell – the platelet – can be suppressed, causing a condition known as idiopathic thrombocytopenic purpura. The risk of developing this condition after receiving the MMR vaccine is much less than the risk of developing it after catching the measles, mumps or rubella infections themselves. For this condition, the balance of risk and benefit is heavily weighted in favour of the vaccine.

The advantages of the MMR vaccine when compared with single vaccines are two-fold. First, vaccine administration is simplified. It is plain that giving three vaccines in one single preparation is an important efficiency improvement for both the child and the family (less pain for the child and less disruption to normal routines for parents). Second, the cost savings are huge. In the US, for example, the net saving gained by using MMR was about $60 million annually compared with using no vaccines at all. Given that all the early evidence showed that MMR had an efficacy and safety profile comparable with single vaccines, the triple vaccine was seen as a massive step forward for child health protection.

If one goes back to read the initial studies of MMR,[5] one sees serious and considered efforts to be sure of safety. Sometimes this earlier preoccupation with safety is not emphasized by those critical of the MMR vaccine today. In one report by Finnish scientists, based on data from 581 twin-pairs, the rate of adverse reactions to the MMR vaccine was between 0.5 per cent and 4 per cent. The commonest side-effects were 'irritability', mild-to-moderate fever and drowsiness. Heikki Peltola and Olli Heinonen were careful in their interpretation of these higher rates of unusual behaviours. They wrote:

> A temporal association between vaccination and symptoms appearing in the following days or weeks does not necessarily imply a causal relationship . . . if a child has been immunized, the parents observe him, intentionally or not, more closely than usual, and will tend to blame the vaccination for any signs or symptoms.

This statement hangs presciently as a comment over the more recent claims by Andrew Wakefield. There was a particular interest during the 1980s in the risk of neurological complications, such as encephalitis. Although a few cases of encephalitis were reported after vaccination, it seemed reasonable to conclude that these cases occurred after vaccination by chance only. One report did describe a vaccine strain of measles in the cerebrospinal fluid of a child who had developed encephalitis,[6] but that was in 1967 and nothing has been reported since. There have been other associations made between live attenuated measles vaccines, including the MMR vaccine, and neurological diseases, but again whether these events were actually related to the vaccine or signified instead only chance associations was and remains impossible to tell.

This is not to say that the MMR vaccine has not had its difficulties, even before Wakefield became one of its most prominent critics. Sometimes this history is glossed over by public health officials today. For example, the Government's official website devoted to MMR states that:[7]

> By the time the combined MMR vaccines were introduced in the
> UK in 1988 they had already been extensively used worldwide –
> in the USA since the early 1970s, and in Sweden and Finland
> since 1982. This practical experience of giving tens of millions of
> doses of MMR vaccine showed that it was both highly effective
> and very safe before it was introduced in the UK.

This summary of events is incomplete. The Government omits to
say that in September 1992 it announced that two of its three
MMR vaccines – Immravax (manufactured by Merieux UK) and
Pluserix (SmithKlineBeecham) – were to be withdrawn following a
reported association between a particular strain (Urabe) of the
mumps vaccine and cases of aseptic meningitis. (The only remaining vaccine was MMR II.) By the autumn of 1994, there was
widespread fear of a resurgent measles epidemic, and so a
measles–rubella vaccination campaign was launched. Priorix was
finally introduced in 1997.

There is an important lesson here in understanding the
strengths and weaknesses of clinical trials. A clinical trial, in which
treatments are randomly allocated to patients, is the best means
scientists have of establishing the efficacy of a new intervention, be
it a drug, a device, or anything else intended to improve the outcome for the patient. But trials are usually a poor way to prove
safety. For example, in one trial Pluserix and MMR II were studied in 174 Finnish children by Timo Vesikari and his colleagues.[8]
There was a high protective response rate to MMR II and Pluserix
(over 95 per cent) for all three infectious diseases. Adverse reactions were also recorded in this study. Recall that Pluserix went on
to be withdrawn, while MMR II remains available to this day. The
only adverse reactions that were more common in children receiving Pluserix were vomiting and local redness at the site of

injection. The risks of Pluserix were missed in these small clinical trials.

The story of the more recent concerns over the MMR vaccine began a long time before the 1998 *Lancet* paper. Almost ten years earlier, Andrew Wakefield was once again the chief protagonist in another intense controversy, and the *Lancet* was his foil. He and his colleagues at the Royal Free Hospital described what they believed to be clues to the cause of a puzzling inflammatory condition of the bowel – Crohn's disease.[9] Wakefield's idea was that the normal blood supply to the gut was compromised, producing local damage (infarction) of the delicate tissues making up the bowel wall. He believed that the discovery of this underlying pathology would clear a path 'to identify a primary causative agent in Crohn's disease'. But what was this causative agent?

I was working at the Royal Free when Wakefield's *Lancet* paper was first published in 1989. I was in a different department to Wakefield, but close enough (we worked at opposite ends of the tenth floor of the hospital) to see the sensation his work caused. Research in the Royal Free's Academic Department of Medicine was largely moribund at the time I was there. The unit's reputation still rested on the brilliantly illustrious career of Dame Sheila Sherlock, Britain's foremost expert on liver disease, who had an international reputation second to none. By 1989, the bars of Belsize Park were rather better filled with medical school research staff than its laboratories. Wakefield brought a sudden sense of excitement to the department. He was young, charismatic, and ambitious. The department felt alive again.

Wakefield's attention turned to measles. He quickly focused on the measles virus as a potential cause of Crohn's disease, both in the laboratory[10] and in epidemiological studies.[11] He eventually suggested that one source of measles might be the measles vaccine. The risk of developing Crohn's disease in those who received live measles vaccine was three times greater than those who did not. Wakefield and his Royal Free colleagues concluded that 'measles virus may play a part' in causing inflammatory bowel disease.[12] They were careful to note that they had not proved cause and effect.

And then in 1998 came the paper reporting a new syndrome of bowel disease and autism in twelve children referred by parents and their doctors to the Royal Free Hospital.[13] When families were asked if they had noticed any particular event prior to the onset of their child's symptoms, two said none, one reported an ear infection, another thought of measles, and eight said the MMR vaccine. 'We did not prove an association,' Wakefield wrote, once again. We editors tried to highlight the preliminary nature of these findings by publishing the article as an 'Early Report'. We also tried to remind readers of the vast global benefits of measles vaccination. We published figures showing that existing measles vaccines had reduced the number of cases of infection by almost 100 per cent, and had cut the annual number of cases in the US alone from 900,000 in 1941 to just 135 in 1997. Two respected vaccine experts, Robert T. Chen and Frank DeStefano from the US Centers for Disease Control and Prevention, invited readers to examine the Wakefield data 'with an open mind'.[14] But they obviously doubted the possibility of the alleged association. Proof would have to await 'critical virological studies', they wrote. Chen and DeStefano also warned that reports such as Wakefield's 'may snowball into societal tragedies when the media and the public confuse association with causality and shun immunization'. The Wakefield paper was the beginning of a sequence of events that saw their concern become a reality.

In the week of the paper's publication, some of the Royal Free research team decided to hold a press conference to announce their findings. This gave them an opportunity to stress the benefits of the MMR vaccine and the inconclusive nature of their results with respect to the link between the syndrome and the vaccine. But even though the event was chaired by Arie Zuckerman, the dean of the medical school where Wakefield worked and a noted vaccine expert himself, the press conference did far more harm than good. Instead of avoiding any unfounded speculations about the safety of the triple vaccine, the team's press release said:

> The majority opinion among the researchers involved in this study supports the continuation of MMR vaccination. Dr Wakefield feels that vaccination against the measles, mumps, and rubella infections should undoubtedly continue but until this issue is resolved by further research there is a case for separating the three vaccines into separate measles, mumps, and rubella components and giving them individually spaced by at least 1 year.

An accompanying Royal Free Hospital video news release opened with a child being vaccinated. Since the vaccine's three components were not available separately in the UK, Wakefield's advice at the press conference was taken, for all practical purposes, as a recommendation to parents not to have their children vaccinated at all until individual vaccines were obtainable. Despite the clear caveats in the research paper, by suggesting that MMR should be divided into its separate vaccines, Wakefield implied that any link between the vaccine and the new syndrome was far stronger than it really was.

His paper – and especially his claims about the safety of the MMR vaccine – unleashed a tidal wave of new research, which continues to this day. The first foundation of a systematic effort to investigate the

Wakefield hypothesis was laid down quickly: it seemed to disprove any link between the MMR vaccine and autism.[15]

That early work was soon corroborated. The key hypothesis – that the MMR vaccine might be an environmental trigger for autism – was refuted, at least in large population studies.[16] Indeed, by June 1999 it was clear from separate Finnish and British studies that there was nothing substantive behind Wakefield's theory. Yet the difficulty remained, and this was conceded by even the most ardent MMR vaccine advocates, that it was almost impossible to rule out a risk altogether. As Brent Taylor wrote in the *Lancet*, his own research did 'not rule out the possibility of a rare idiosyncratic response to MMR'. Nevertheless, he was surely right to argue that his 'results will reassure parents and others who have been concerned about the possibility that MMR vaccine is likely to cause autism'.

Since these initial negative reports, repeated studies in many different settings have supported the safety of the MMR vaccine – in a UK database of patients run by general practitioners, in a group of Californian children born between 1980 and 1994, in children living in North London, in over 500,000 Finnish children aged one to seven, in over 400,000 Danish children who had received the MMR vaccine, and in children living in metropolitan Atlanta.[17]

Nevertheless, several curious facts emerged from these reports. There remained no clear explanation for the well-documented increase in recorded diagnoses of autism (I discuss this conundrum further in Chapter 4). There was no evidence to compare and contrast the risks of the triple MMR vaccine with single vaccines. There was evidence that parental histories changed after Wakefield's findings became public.[18] Before that point, families noted concerns about their child's health early in his or her life. After the MMR furore, they pinpointed their child's illness to a time after MMR vaccination. Scientists call this kind of altered testimony 'recall bias'. It means that any study relying on remembered events recalled by a parent or a patient (and even a doctor) should be treated with caution, even scepticism. And finally, the need for continuous surveillance of vaccine safety to differentiate between chance occurrences and true adverse events was frequently emphasized, despite the absence of a link with autism.

Meanwhile, Wakefield and several other research teams began to report laboratory, as opposed to epidemiological, evidence to support their theory that measles was somehow linked to autism.[19] In collaboration with a Japanese group, Wakefield reported the presence of measles virus in some patients with chronic bowel disease. In nine children with the autism–bowel syndrome, now labelled as 'autistic enterocolitis', three were positive for measles and Wakefield claimed that the measles virus he found was 'consistent with being vaccine' related.

Another research group at Utah State University, led by Vijendra Singh, described the existence of what he called an 'unusual' MMR antibody in almost two-thirds of a sample of children with autism (seventy-five of 125 children). The antibody was not detected in a group of non-autistic children. The beginnings of a mechanism behind an MMR vaccine link to autism were now being teased out – allegedly. Singh argued that 'it seems plausible that autistic children elicited an inappropriate or abnormal antibody response to MMR'. He speculated that these children had 'faulty' immune systems and concluded that 'It is quite possible that vaccines in a small population of genetically predisposed children may react inappropriately, simply because of their immature immune system or some other unknown factors.' Singh went on to study a further eighty-eight autistic children and found that their levels of measles antibody were significantly higher than children without autism. He interpreted these findings as suggesting a causal role for measles virus in autism. Could it be that these children were displaying an abnormal immune reaction to the vaccine?[20]

There was a clear disparity in the evidence. Epidemiology showed that the MMR vaccine had absolutely no relation to autism. Even Wakefield's own research showed this fact to be true.[21] But what he and others were seeing in the laboratory pointed to a quite different conclusion. It seemed fair to argue that if the MMR vaccine was mostly safe, there remained a small possibility that it was causing a syndrome of autistic enterocolitis in a very small number of children. Yet was this new syndrome itself real or apparent?

After the 1998 *Lancet* paper was published, a quite separate line of research was established to explore the nature of this apparently new constellation of symptoms and signs.[22] These studies did seem to show that children with autism sometimes had disorders of the gastrointestinal tract that had hitherto gone unrecognized, such as inflammation of the oesophagus, stomach and upper intestine. These conditions may have been contributing to the behavioural changes that children were experiencing.

After publication of the original *Lancet* paper describing the first twelve children with autistic enterocolitis seen at the Royal Free Hospital, a further sixty children were reported two years later. The results from these children confirmed and extended the earlier findings. More detailed laboratory investigations of these subtle gut lesions revealed the true nature of the inflammatory disease of the bowel – there seemed to be a disruption to the normal workings of the lining of the intestine. Wakefield and his colleagues proposed that the pathology they were seeing in the gut was somehow linked to the pathology to be found in the brain. Was some kind of immune disease the connection between the two phenomena? Wakefield urged further research, especially clinical trials of possible new treatments. This research was important because 'desperate parents will understandably seek whatever may possibly help, and with modern communications, are exposed to a bewildering array of unvalidated claims'. These were wise words. Regrettably, he did not have them to mind in 1998 when he advocated splitting the MMR vaccine on the grounds of similarly unvalidated claims.

In December 2001, the UK's Medical Research Council (MRC) released an important report summarizing the state of our knowledge about the causes of autism.[23] Their analysis included an appraisal of the so-called syndrome of autistic enterocolitis. The MRC was anxious about the possibility that the children studied by Wakefield were part of a biased sample. That is, they did not accurately represent the vast majority of children with autism, but instead reflected the selection of a very particular subgroup of these children, a subgroup whose parents knew of Wakefield's interest in the MMR vaccine. In sum, the MRC concluded that although this work was 'interesting and in principle worth investigating', better research methods and independent replication were 'crucial' if these preliminary reports were to become accepted mainstream thinking.

The Royal Free research team has continued to publish work looking at the molecular mechanisms that might underpin their earlier findings.[24] In collaboration with John O'Leary in Dublin, Wakefield believed that he had found evidence of measles virus in the intestinal tissue of these children. In 2002, they claimed that they had, for the very first time, linked measles virus directly with autistic enterocolitis. Wakefield and his team went on to show that children with this type of autism had an entirely new kind of bowel disease that was suggestive of an immune system attacking its own tissues – autoimmunity.

The difficulty for Wakefield, who left the Royal Free Hospital in 2002 voluntarily but under considerable pressure, is that no other research group has published work fully confirming his own findings. There have been hints of confirmation. For example, Dr Tim Buie, a paediatric gastroenterologist at the Massachusetts General Hospital in America, has found that a substantial number of children – around half of those he has examined – have treatable gastrointestinal problems, including enterocolitis and lymphoid nodular hyperplasia. Buie is quoted on the website of the Northwestern United States Autism Foundation as saying that, 'These children are ill, in distress and pain, and not just mentally, neurologically dysfunctional.' This site carries insignias for both Harvard Medical School and MassGeneral Hospital for Children, indicating its respectability and authority. But, as yet, Buie's findings remain unpublished.

Without independent replication, as the MRC report has pointed out, Wakefield's work carries far less persuasive weight. Some reports, such as those by Sydney Finegold in Los Angeles and Magee DeFelice in Philadelphia, have pointed to some unusual observations in children with autism. Finegold, for example, discovered abnormal patterns of bacterial colonization in the intestines of autistic children. DeFelice found differences between children with and without autism in a group of chemicals that can drive inflammation. But he concluded that his results 'failed to support' a causal link between autism and bowel disease.

The research into bowel disease and autism has continued at the Royal Free Hospital without Wakefield, among a team led by Simon Murch – the hospital's senior paediatric gastroenterologist. His group has discovered distinctive patterns of inflammation in the stomachs of children with autism when they are compared with children who have Crohn's disease, children who have an infection with the ulcer-causing bacterium *Helicobacter pylori*, and children who are otherwise normal. Murch and his colleagues call the lesion they have discovered 'novel', but also 'subtle'. Its significance is 'uncertain', they say, but could have 'therapeutic relevance'. At the very least, they 'suggest that the pediatric gastroenterologist may play a valid role in the global assessment of the child with autism'. It remains entirely possible that autism is a condition that affects many body systems, not only the brain. This potential profound complexity deserves serious scientific attention, not angry dismissal.

Those who remain sceptical of the MMR vaccine's safety, despite an apparently overwhelming body of evidence to the contrary, are unlikely to withdraw from this field of debate admitting defeat. In 2000, a charity called Visceral was launched under the rather frightening strapline, 'Something strange is happening to young children. . .' Visceral's website sets out its goals very clearly:

> Visceral is the only charity in the UK, and one of a handful of charities in the US, that coordinates and funds research into the relationship between environmental factors and the recent increases in diagnoses of autism that have occurred in many developed world countries. Visceral's research programme is directed by Andrew Wakefield FRCS FRCPath, who is the charity's full-time Chief Medical Scientist. The principal hypotheses under investigation at present concern an association between measles containing vaccines and children with regressive autism and an inflammatory bowel disease.

In 2004, the charity claimed to be funding at least thirty-five scientists doing sixteen studies in medical schools and research institutes across America and Europe. Visceral described itself as being 'the leading organization supporting research into the gastrointestinal disorders that often occur in conjunction with regressive autism'. It called attention to its three-year research programme, which it estimated would cost US $6.5 million, 'a comparatively small sum that could help hundreds of thousands of people affected by these chronic gastrointestinal diseases'.

The future directions of the anti-MMR vaccine campaigners were outlined in February 2004 at a meeting of the Immunization Safety Review Committee of the Institute of Medicine, held at the US National Academy of Sciences in Washington, DC. The Institute of Medicine was conducting its own investigation into vaccines and autism. One presentation was co-written by Andrew Wakefield, who described himself as Director of Research at the International Child Development Resource Center. The ICDRC is part of an organization called the Good News Doctor Foundation, whose logo is a stethoscope sitting on top of a bible. Located in Melbourne, Florida, the Foundation describes itself as: 'A Christian ministry that provides hope and information on how to eat better, feel better, and minister more effectively as a result of a biblically based, healthy lifestyle.' It is led by two physicians, Dr Jeff Bradstreet, a co-author with Wakefield of the February 2004 presentation to the Institute of Medicine, and Dr Jerold J. Kartzinel, whose biography notes that his youngest son 'has autism which developed after his 15th month MMR immunization'.

As in the UK, Wakefield and Bradstreet presented themselves as doctors who listened to parents when 'oftentimes the profession met them with scepticism and dismissed their concerns'. One strand of their research involved what they proposed was a 'pattern of public deception' concerning a mercury-based vaccine preservative, thimerosal, and autism. They argued that there were 'elevated relative burdens' of mercury in children with autistic spectrum disorders and that there was a 'definable genomic and biochemical abnormality' in these children that 'would make them potentially more vulnerable to mercury exposure'.

A second strand of their work concerned the MMR vaccine. Wakefield and Bradstreet told the Immunization Safety Review Committee that they had confirmed evidence of actively replicating measles virus in the bowel, blood and cerebrospinal fluid of children with autistic spectrum disorders. They claimed that when autism was suspected, the measles strain was 'always of vaccine origin'. Very little of this work has been published in peer-reviewed scientific journals.

And while this public debate continues, despite a retraction of the interpretation concerning the MMR vaccine and autism, health warnings about the consequences of not having an adequately immunized population are persistently repeated.[25] General practitioners were struggling throughout 2004 to encourage parents to adopt the vaccine. Here are extracts from one particularly pleading letter to parents from two GPs working in the south of England:

From our point of view we have had no problems, at any stage, from any one single MMR vaccination. There are three autistic children in the practice, two of whom have not had the MMR vaccination, and one who has. We have no young children in the practice with any bowel disorders under the age of about 15. The only reactions we have had are local skin reactions, slight red swelling, a feeling of being unwell for maybe a couple of days, occasional vague temperature for a couple of days, but certainly no significant reactions. This is counterbalanced against our own experience of doctors in the 'old days', when [one of us] has seen measles encephalitis on two occasions. In South Africa, where he worked on his student elective, 15% of the Zulu population died from measles. . . Dr — has had all his children vaccinated, as appropriate . . . Those who are not vaccinated are depending upon the herd immunity from those who have been vaccinated, to keep the general number of cases of measles, mumps, and rubella down . . . We realize that not everybody will have the vaccination done for their children, but we hope that you will reconsider your stand on the issue . . .'

There have also been unfortunate occasions where an enthusiasm to immunize has overridden the wishes of parents, forcing embarrassing public apologies. In May 2004 a Leeds schoolgirl was given the MMR vaccine despite her parents signing two forms exempting her from immunization. In this instance, the parents were uncertain about the safety of the vaccine. Leeds health authorities admitted their 'regrettable mistake', apologized, and emphasized that they supported the right of parents to choose or refuse immunization. In another even more egregious example, it took the intervention of a primary care trust to reverse the decision of a general practice in London which had threatened to deregister an entire family for deciding not to have their daughter vaccinated. For some doctors, vaccination is not about altruism, it is about coercion.

So, is the MMR vaccine safe or not? Looked at on a panoramic, population scale, the answer is clearly yes. Multiple epidemiological studies, completed in different geographical locations by different investigators, have found no evidence for any association between the MMR vaccine and autism.

The frequently voiced objection to this view is that the vaccine is exerting its damaging effects in a small group of susceptible children. The numbers of children affected are too small to be picked up by crude epidemiological surveys, these critics argue. MMR vaccine advocates have four objections to this claim. First, that any formulation of a coherent hypothesis against the vaccine is hopelessly weak, depending as it does on fragmentary, unpublished data that amount to little more than speculation. Second, that what weak laboratory evidence does exist is almost always linked in some way to Andrew Wakefield. There remains no believable alternative source of evidence – a simple, straightforward, and peer-reviewed replication would do – to support Wakefield's contentions.

Two further defences have been advanced, both of which are powerful but also sometimes counter-productive. One concerns the characteristics of the individuals involved. Most scientists conduct their public disputes openly and directly with their opponents. Wakefield conducts some of his exchanges through the hands of a public relations company, Bell Pottinger. Wakefield is now also the Director of Research and Chief Medical Scientist for two organizations that have adopted the MMR vaccine theory of autism as one of their central campaigning issues, and whose future depends upon direct solicitation of money from the public to fund their activities. An ungenerous view of these arrangements might be that it is hard to maintain a reputation for scientific neutrality when the funding of the research one is doing depends on marketing a message of acute anxiety – even despair – to parents of children with autism. Advancing a message of safety and reassurance would hardly keep the money rolling in. Supporters of Wakefield would say that such a view is part of the well-managed witch-hunt against him. But there surely is a difficulty here. Whatever Wakefield's positive qualities, he has repeatedly put himself in positions that allow his enemies to question his motives.

A second (and very dangerous) defence is that even if there was a tiny risk attached to the MMR vaccine,[26] the burden of illness related to measles, mumps and rubella infections is sufficiently large and so easily prevented by the vaccine that in any reasonable calculus of risk and benefit, the vaccine always wins. This is not an argument that has ever been advanced by the UK's Department of Health, and it is one for which no evidence of such a tiny risk has been produced in order to support it. Still, this point has been made by doctors who feel that the logical impossibility of proving a negative (that the MMR vaccine does not cause autism) is so damaging that even a desperate calculus of risk and benefit is preferable to offering no rational defence for immunization at all.

The totality of available evidence should certainly assure parents that the MMR vaccine is not a cause of autism or the bowel disorder known as autistic enterocolitis. This conclusion has been reached by every research study and authoritative body that has considered the matter, including those independent of government and those in medicine without any vested interest in arguing in favour of the vaccine.[27] Andrew Wakefield disputes this consensus. Writing in the *Lancet* in response to the retraction published by his colleagues, he argued that despite the debate surrounding his February 1998 *Lancet* paper, 'It would be inappropriate to interpret the events of the past month as exonerating MMR vaccine as a possible cause of autism.'[28]

But Wakefield's position received a further blow in May 2004, when the Institute of Medicine, America's lead agency for providing scientific advice on matters of health and medicine, published its final report on vaccines and autism. The Institute's eleven-member committee had the benefit of reviewing the events leading up to the retraction of the interpretation in the *Lancet*. After an incredibly rigorous evaluation of all the available data, the committee concluded that 'the evidence favours rejection of a causal relationship between MMR vaccine and autism'. Any hypothesis connecting the vaccine to autism was 'theoretical only'. In the light of this conclusion, they recommended that there should be no policy review of the licensing of the MMR vaccine. The report had particular value because the members of the panel selected by the Institute of Medicine to review the evidence were chosen according to strict criteria – namely, that they had neither links to vaccine manufacturers nor any association with ongoing vaccine litigation. Their conclusions were as unbiased as one was ever likely to get.

Rather perversely, the security of this judgement was inadvertently questioned by Professor Jean Golding from the University of Bristol. In May 2004, she was awarded a £400,000 grant by the UK's Medical Research Council (MRC) to study the role of environmental risks in the development of autism. The risks that the MRC had in mind were infections in the mother and fetus, exposure to chemical toxins, diet and problems with the birth of the child. One might have thought that the question of the MMR vaccine, given the weight of evidence gathered so far, would not have been a serious issue in this research. But in an interview on Britain's *Today* programme on BBC Radio 4, Golding seemed to cast fresh doubt on the vaccine's safety by suggesting, perhaps by accident, that she was approaching the issue of the MMR vaccine's supposed link to autism with 'an open mind'. Here is the exchange Golding had with John Humphrys:

JOHN HUMPHRYS: . . . your working hypothesis to the extent that you have one is that it's what a mother does during pregnancy is likely to determine [autism]?

JEAN GOLDING: That's . . . that's certainly what I feel but we will look at all other features that have happened after the baby was born as well.

JOHN HUMPHRYS: Including MMR?

JEAN GOLDING: Including MMR, yes.

JOHN HUMPHRYS: Do you have a view on that at the moment?

JEAN GOLDING: Well, all the evidence that has taken a large number of children and looked for a MMR association has failed to find it. So I doubt whether we're going to find anything but we will certainly look with an open mind.

JOHN HUMPHRYS: That's . . . that's the important thing isn't it, that you do have an open mind on this because there are many people who say that the scientific community has closed its mind to the possibility.

JEAN GOLDING: No we certainly haven't.

If I were a parent listening to this discussion, I think that I would have been left more, not less, confused about the safety of the vaccine. It sounded like a truly definitive answer would have to await even more research. Indeed, despite the *Lancet's* retraction of Wakefield's published interpretation concerning his 1998 findings, there remains continuing public, although not scientific, uncertainty about the safety of the MMR vaccine. Outbreaks of measles are occurring sporadically across Britain – in south Wales, for example, in July 2004, as a consequence of a children's party and at a time of only 70 per cent vaccine coverage in the Swansea area.

Some observers point out that, given what they see as this residual uncertainty about the safety of the MMR vaccine, single vaccines should be made more widely available to parents through the National Health Service. This view has support in some surprising quarters. In April 2004, for example, I spoke with one professor of medicine who is also an administrator in a well-known Royal College. He told me, with a note of defiance in his voice, that he still recommended the single measles vaccine to parents of children that he saw in his clinic. Yet single vaccinations of each measles, mumps and rubella component would involve six injections instead of two. The widespread use of three single vaccines has never been tested, whereas MMR has been subjected to several trials of clinical effectiveness. From what doctors know about these vaccines, the likelihood is that full protection against all three diseases could take as long as five years, well beyond the government's quite reasonable and responsible target of pre-school protection against measles, mumps and rubella. This risk would be increased by the possibility that at least some of the six injections would be missed.

Finally, what lessons are to be learned from the MMR vaccine debate for future vaccines and vaccination campaigns? This is not a question that many doctors, especially those within Britain's Department of Health or public health establishment, want to answer – at least in public. And one can understand why. In a review of the unintended effects associated with the MMR vaccine, Tom Jefferson and his colleagues, on behalf of the European Research Program for Improved Vaccine Safety Surveillance Project, found that the reporting of safety outcomes in MMR vaccine studies was inadequate.[29]

Here is a frequently repeated scenario in health-technology assessment. A product undergoes limited clinical testing for efficacy and safety. A signal of concern is thrown up. There is no valid set of safety data to which one can turn in order to answer these queries. Public concern grows and confidence in the technology may be jeopardized. Appropriate studies are hastily completed to confirm or refute the original signal of potential risk. An answer eventually comes, but too late to prevent a great deal of unnecessary anxiety. And in the case of the MMR vaccine, real harm. Measles outbreaks are now occurring in areas where vaccine uptake is low – in one especially upsetting instance, causing encephalitis among children who had undergone kidney transplants.[30]

Jefferson has proposed a solution to this recurring problem. His idea is to create a 'library of evidence' within the Department of Health, drawing together widely dispersed data from published papers, vaccine manufacturers' technical reports and investigators' personal files. In this way, loss of crucial information would be kept to a minimum and gaps in the existing evidence could be identified and filled early on.[31] His idea has been rejected by medical authorities. 'It won't do the job,' I was told by one informed Department of Health adviser. Officials seem understandably frightened to admit that the safeguards they had in place to protect confidence in the MMR vaccine were threadbare. And they seem too complacent, now that Wakefield's theory is all but discredited, to grapple with ways to implement Jefferson's ingenious idea to prevent a similar public health disaster in the future. For happen again it surely will.

Indeed, we have been in exactly this position once before.[32] In the 1980s, many parents in America began to ask questions about the safety of vaccines, in much the same way that parents in Britain today express concerns about the MMR vaccine. The anxieties in the US were so great that parents stopped getting their children immunized. Vaccine manufacturers even threatened to pull out of vaccine production altogether because of escalating litigation. In response, Congress passed the National Childhood Vaccine Injury Act in 1986. This legislation led to a review by the Institute of Medicine of the evidence surrounding the alleged links between vaccines, including the MMR vaccine, and subsequent illnesses. No system existed at the time to resolve these concerns routinely. A committee of vaccine experts, together with scientists who understood the criteria that needed to be satisfied in order to prove cause and effect, conducted an eighteen month investigation. They scoured electronic databases for evidence of vaccine-related adverse events. They searched their own extensive personal files of scientific literature. And they analysed over 500 unpublished case reports that had accumulated randomly over the years and which may have thrown additional light on whether a particular vaccine was harmful or not.

After reviewing all the evidence they could lay their hands on, and after listening to testimony from scientists as well as parents of allegedly vaccine-damaged children, they published their report in 1993. The committee found that the MMR vaccine was a certain cause of the thrombocytopenia I referred to earlier in this chapter, as well as a very rare type of severe allergic reaction. There had been concerns that the MMR vaccine had somehow caused cases of deafness – but the committee concluded that the evidence was inadequate to accept or reject such a causal relation.

What were the lessons of this episode? The committee expressed dismay that for such an important matter as the safety of childhood vaccinations, they had only case reports and poorly designed research studies to rely on. Reliable estimates of risk should come from carefully conducted epidemiological investigations – of which there were almost none. They recommended four important changes to the way in which vaccines were evaluated for safety. First, disease registries for some of the rarer conditions that might be vaccine-related should be created as one means to study any alleged adverse association in more detail. Second, the effectiveness of the rather informal, passive, and patchy vaccine surveillance system currently in place should be formally investigated. Third, more active surveillance measures should be implemented. And finally, such active surveillance should include formal epidemiological investigations in defined populations where immunization and subsequent clinical care can be properly linked.

In other words, the scare over the MMR vaccine in the UK was entirely preventable. We knew enough in the 1990s, based on the experiences in America, to create a system to protect the credibility of the MMR vaccine should a new signal of risk be thrown up. Instead, our public health system failed. And it could fail once more if an hypothesis such as Wakefield's were ever to surface again.

CHAPTER 2

Science Friction

'The great remedy for slander, just as for troubles in the mind, is time.'

During four weeks in February and March 2004, from the first revelations of alleged impropriety by Andrew Wakefield (his undeclared perceived conflict of interest, among other claims) to the partial retraction of the 1998 *Lancet* paper by the majority of its authors, I carried with me and read repeatedly a short volume of essays called *Justice is Conflict* by Stuart Hampshire.[1] This little book kept the whole affair in perspective during moments of acute doubt and occasional outright fear, as the media's interest intensified all around us.[2] Hampshire's theme is human rationality. According to his simple but compelling test of rationality, public efforts to resolve questions about the safety of the MMR vaccine have failed badly.

Of course, there is nothing especially surprising about this conclusion. The fact that MMR immunization rates have fallen in the face of such weak evidence attests to the apparent irrationality of the human mind – a perplexing and all too humbling observation on twenty-first-century science in society. Yet his modest proposition, if generally agreed, opens up new opportunities to arrange public engagement about controversial matters, especially those rooted in highly specialist and usually closed disciplines such as science.

Hampshire begins *Justice is Conflict* by looking back over his work as a political philosopher. He now rejects, contrary to a lifetime of passionately held views, the notion that there is a universally valid moral theory. There is, sadly, no ideal society to strive for. There are no generalizable principles of social justice. All that can be said is that there exists a set of 'acceptable rational procedures of negotiation'. His 'positive conclusion' – at the end of a life lived during times of violence and atrocity, led by people in the quest for power, and often motivated by hate – was 'to distinguish between justice and fairness in matters of substance and justice and fairness in matters of procedure'. Matters of substance would always vary with different moral outlooks. But 'fairness in procedure is an invariable value, a constant in human nature'. Hampshire's universal principle is simple and it is this: to hear the other side ('audi alteram partem'). Adjudication between conflicting claims demands that society has the right institutions and procedures in place to do so. This should be society's overriding concern.

For Hampshire, human rationality is linked inextricably to justice. The origins of rationality lie in 'the adversary reasoning typical of legal and moral disputes about evidence'. In other words, to be rational means avoiding the intellectual equivalent of the pub brawl. Rationality means establishing the means to achieve procedural fairness – whether the setting is a duel or the law court – so that contrary claims can be heard. Hampshire sees human conflict as inevitable and perpetual. The trick for those seeking a rational society is to manage this conflict 'in conditions of uncertainty'.

The successful oversight of conflict is an urgent matter of species survival, especially in an age of terrorism and political violence.

Instead of reiterating universal declarations of peace and accord, we need to devote more time, according to Hampshire, to protecting and augmenting institutions and procedures that enable all sides in a dispute to be heard. This 'institutionalized fairness' is 'the cement that holds the state together'. Hampshire writes that:

> Rationality is a bond between persons, but it is not a very powerful bond, and it is apt to fail as a bond when there are strong passions on two sides of a conflict. What sentiment can reinforce the bond in a conflict where there are passionate loyalties on both sides? . . . The answer can be found only in institutional loyalties and in deep-seated habits of living together and arguing together.

If we violate this principle, 'we should expect catastrophe'.

The reason why I find this argument so convincing (even comforting) is that however unpleasant the debate about the MMR vaccine became (and becomes), I console myself with Hampshire's view that the extreme adversarial positions that have been staked out and are being defended so aggressively are simply part of this 'norm of rationality'. This statement is not a plea for laissez-faire complacency about the destructive debate surrounding the MMR vaccine. Instead, his portrait of a rational society poses important questions for all of us caught up in this row, whether we are parents or professors, jurists or journalists. Here are some of the questions that, as yet, remain unanswered (and quite possibly unasked).

1. When a debate about a scientific issue (the MMR vaccine, genetically modified foods, and so on) occurs, who are deemed to be acceptable public adversaries worthy of opposing one another? In the case of the MMR vaccine, the

Department of Health, for example, has put too little emphasis on understanding the concerns and views of families with children who have autism. Are those families ruled out as non-expert and therefore inferior protagonists by our politicians and public health officials? If so, why?

2. What precisely is the activity we call 'reasoning'? Are accusatory newspaper headlines, personal attacks, and dismissals of genuinely held beliefs part of what we would reasonably call reasoning? If not, then what does constitute reasoned argument? And if so, then in what sense is this a fair way of arriving at the truth? Or is fairness irrelevant?

3. If we accept that reasoning is our goal in the face of uncertainty, who defines what is uncertain? Who judges the moment at which that uncertainty is resolved? And what is it, anyway, to say that an uncertainty is no longer an uncertainty? If the Department of Health states that there is no uncertainty over the safety of the MMR vaccine, does that negate the uncertainty felt by parents? Or, conversely, if a small group of parents and doctors claim uncertainty about the MMR vaccine, do those claims establish a clear case of doubt that needs to be acknowledged (and so legitimized), investigated, answered, and acted upon, perhaps widening public uncertainty unnecessarily?

4. If we assume that reasoning in the face of uncertainty is taking place, who defines what evidence is admissible to diminish that uncertainty? How is one piece of evidence to be pitted against another? Who decides – and how – whether one bit of evidence wins over another? In other words, what constitutes a victory in any rational argument? Is it a matter of 100 per cent consensus? Or should victory be defined as arriving at an answer beyond all reasonable

doubt (for example, with 99 per cent of the evidence favouring one position or the other), or on the balance of probabilities (such as 51 per cent of the evidence in one direction)? Or should we collectively apply the precautionary principle – accepting that a concern falling well below proof can and should trigger some kind of regulatory intervention, such as the withdrawal of a product or the provision of an alternative?

5. And finally, where is reasoning to be played out? Everywhere, at all times, and in all media? Or should there be, in addition, a more formal space that we endow with special privileges, where reasoning is to be conducted, with rules of evidence, engagement and judgement?

My point is that we have no answers to these urgent questions. And because we have no answers, we are living through a civic crisis of rationality, one that nobody seems willing or able to address, but one that the dispute over the MMR vaccine all too readily underlines. Hampshire ends his book with a disturbing conclusion – namely, that if rationality fails,

> Conflicts will then no longer be resolved within the political domain but will be resolved by violence or the threat of violence . . . whatever one's conception of the good, such anarchy will generally be reckoned a great evil, alongside starvation, and near-starvation, disease, imprisonment, slavery, and humiliation.

When there is only an informal process for public argument, there will be ample room for theorists of conspiracies to make hay. In the midst of allegation and counter-allegation about the probity of Wakefield's research, for example, one newspaper argued that those lined up against his work were part of a 'transparently orchestrated campaign'.[3] The case against us was that the Royal Free Hospital, the Chief Medical Officer, ministers (including the Prime Minister and presumably his son Leo), the *Sunday Times*, a Liberal Democrat MP and possibly every public health official in the country had somehow colluded to urge parents to ignore Wakefield's conclusions. The editors of the *Independent* called for 'a thorough scientific debate' to neutralize the Government's supposedly untrustworthy reassurances.

Yet behind the scenes of this public furore, there was little harmony among these disparate parties, many of whom were competing for position (and sometimes reputation) in an atmosphere of barely concealed mutual loathing. And it all became extremely personal. I received a letter from British Telecom, for example, dated 21 February 2004, the day after we released our statement concerning the allegations made against the Royal Free research team, apologizing for being unable to answer my queries. BT believed that I had called them three times asking for details of my home telephone account. They refused to pass on any information since I could not quote my BT account number. They could not be sure, they wrote, that I was an authorized caller. And, indeed, 'I' was not. Whoever had called BT was not me – it was somebody impersonating me, presumably to discover to whom I was making private telephone calls. Who might I have been calling? Andrew Wakefield? Liam Donaldson? John Reid? Leo Blair? None of these, in fact. But indulging in the criminal offence of trying to gain access to personal telephone records by deception was hardly the behaviour of a collegial group of orchestrated conspirators. The disagreements among friends and colleagues sometimes became acute. On the morning of 21 February I was interviewed by John Humphrys on Radio 4's *Today* programme. I was asked whether MMR was safe. I could, and probably should, have said that, given the available evidence, as far as anyone could tell the vaccine was, indeed, safe. What I actually said was something quite different:

JOHN HUMPHRYS: In very simple terms, do you believe the MMR jab is safe?
ME: Absolutely safe.
JOHN HUMPHRYS: [*clearly incredulous*] Absolutely safe?
ME: Absolutely safe. So much safe that our own three-year-old daughter has had MMR and is extremely well and is protected, and is contributing to community protection against these three infectious diseases.

That exchange triggered an email from a very senior and knighted doctor, a friend whom I have long respected and admired, but who felt that I had been extremely foolish in my choice of words. He wrote, 'Richard, by insisting that MMR is absolutely safe I think that you encourage a widespread and mistaken belief that science can prove negatives. Forgive me, but it's a John Selwyn Gummer type of mistake, and a hostage to fortune, if only because it's so easily challenged in logic.'

It wasn't the charge of illogicality that upset me. Public health messages inevitably eliminate complex disagreements over evidence in order to convey a simpler picture, fairly I think, of what the majority of doctors and experts believe to be true, according to the best of their knowledge. What really stung, and still does, was equating my decision to mention my three-year-old daughter's experience with MMR with John Selwyn Gummer's attempt to end concern about the safety of British beef by forcing a hamburger into the mouth of his daughter at the height of the crisis over bovine spongiform encephalopathy. I could see the point of my friend's criticism, although I felt the circumstances were different. I was, after all, reporting a fact – my daughter's vaccination – that had taken place over a year before. I was not administering the vaccine live on air.

These personal frictions were quickly superseded by more threatening challenges. The GMC sent a team from its Manchester offices to begin assembling evidence in London. John Reid had urged the Council to investigate Wakefield and the allegations made against him of research misconduct. And the newspaper that had first launched an investigation into the original work on autism and the MMR vaccine was continuing its inquiries.

These inquiries had become marred by a disagreement between Brian Deer, the investigative journalist leading the *Sunday Times* investigations, and myself. Deer and I differed about the circumstances of his visit to the *Lancet* on 18 February 2004. He threatened to refer me to the Press Complaints Commission, to file a complaint against my employers, to investigate my position with regard to other editors in order to ascertain their reaction to my conduct, and to take me to court for loss of earnings. Among other things, he also accused me of indulging in a 'readership-building controversy' and of being 'an old Royal Free chum' of Andrew Wakefield. The headline that appeared on his website (briandeer.com) summarized his view of me: 'Whitewashed by the *Lancet*?'

One place where controlled conflict can take place is Parliament. Political interest in the disclosures over the Royal Free research began with a Liberal Democrat MP. Shortly after we released our statement on 20 February regarding the allegations against Wakefield and his colleagues, Evan Harris tabled a written question to John Reid asking, 'How has he satisfied himself that lumbar punctures carried out on children at the Royal Free Hospital by the inflammatory bowel disease study group since 1996 have had valid and effective ethical approval from a properly constituted ethical committee, on the basis of the researchers' relevant interests and the full clinical context?'

But the politics were not straightforward. The House of Commons Science and Technology Committee, chaired by Dr Ian Gibson MP, and on which Evan Harris also sat, was in the middle of an inquiry into scientific publications. The committee's investigation had been driven by a long-running argument over access to scientific information. The *Lancet* is owned by Reed-Elsevier, one of the world's largest international medical and scientific publishers. Reed-Elsevier's chief executive officer, Crispin Davis, was due to give evidence before Gibson's committee on 1 March 2004. The MMR vaccine issue was bound to come up, and the *Lancet* was likely to be a target for the committee's questioning. I had not talked with Crispin Davis directly. In truth, I was somewhat nervous about what he might say. The issue was a complex one even for those of us dealing with it day-to-day. The details of ethics committee approvals, subgroups of children with autism, invasive medical investigations, pathologies of bowel disease, and the nuances of conflicts of interest all provided opportunities to be tripped up, especially by politicians searching for inconsistencies in the evidence.[4] In the event, the *Lancet* and its role in Wakefield's work did exercise the committee. The first question from Robert Key MP was little more than a gentle provocation.

MR KEY: Mr Davis, your company owns the *Lancet*. Do you think that scientific publishers have a responsibility towards society to ensure that the research they publish is authenticated and not affected by conflict of interest?

MR DAVIS: We absolutely have a responsibility to ensure that what we publish is peer reviewed, accurate, reflects best practice. In the issue of the *Lancet* we do have a policy where people who submit their articles have to declare any conflict of interest. You can imagine that it is virtually impossible for every editor to research every single author in terms of conflict of interest, and in this one Dr Wakefield said there was no conflict of interest, and in fact three months later in written form repeated that there was no conflict of interest. In all fairness, I do not hold our editor to blame in that instance. I think it was regrettable but I do not think he or the *Lancet* were at fault at all. We were in our opinion badly misled.

After a digression into the realms of pharmaceutical industry influences in medical research, Evan Harris returned to the *Lancet*:

DR HARRIS: Coming back to this issue of Dr Wakefield, I am conscious of the fact that it is a force for editorial freedom for proprietors, and you have given a view. Is it consistent to say that you feel you did not have full disclosure and indeed, three months later, following an allegation in the letters page, there was a specific denial, and then your editor said that the article was fatally flawed? Should that not be equivalent to a retraction rather than a correcting editorial under the code guidelines, or are you happy that that is where we are at?

MR DAVIS: I am not happy that this is where we are at at all, for obvious reasons, but I think that the editor behaved in absolutely the right way. At the time of the submission of the article there was no admission of conflict of interest. Three months later there was a written letter. I think I have got it somewhere here.

DR HARRIS: I have it as well, 7 May 1998 [the letter was actually dated 2 May 1998].

MR DAVIS: It actually says, 'There is no conflict of interest.' Should the editor then—

DR HARRIS: I am talking about now. Now it has come to light why did this not get retracted, particularly given that the conflict of interest has been said to go to the core of one of the scientific findings of the paper, that there was a link between MMR and autism and because there is a legal case going on with four of the patients?

MR DAVIS: I think the editor did immediately, when this was brought to his attention, say publicly that the research therefore was – I think the words he used were – fatally flawed.

DR HARRIS: Why is that not a retraction? Why is the article not being retracted or are you happy not to have your editors retract articles that are fatally flawed?

MR JONGEJAN [a senior colleague of Crispin Davis]: To my knowledge the editor is not excluding at this point that this is the end of the investigation by himself or by any other party, so I think this issue is in that sense still open.

As Arie Jongejan had hinted, we were already working on the terms of a partial retraction. When that came two days later, on 3 March, members of the Science and Technology Committee erupted in anger. Gibson called for the 1998 *Lancet* article by Wakefield to be retracted in full.[5] He said, 'There can be no such thing as a partial retraction. You either believe in your data or you don't.' He claimed that our actions did us 'no credit'. Harris described our position as a 'nonsense'. He called for a full public inquiry (again). Of the *Lancet*, Gibson said, 'Yes, they are on the line, he [that is, I was] on the line, his editorial board is on the line and I look forward to his reply to his [*sic*] questions.'

These questions came in a letter from the Science and

Technology Committee several days later.[6] The rather threatening earlier rhetoric had now given way to a series of fair and forensic questions, none of them referring explicitly to the MMR vaccine or the Wakefield paper itself. I was asked to explain how the *Lancet* ensured the integrity of our peer-review process. I was invited to describe how the journal took responsibility for research papers after publication – 'for example, in deciding to publish a paper, what weight is attached to the possibility that certain campaigners are likely to attach an exaggerated significance to certain papers which support their view?' I was also asked to 'outline' our policy on retraction and to explain the nature of partial retraction.[7]

The temperature of our disagreement rose steeply a few days later. On 4 March, Harris called for and won time to debate what he described as 'the outrageous activities that have been taking place at the Royal Free Hospital since 1995'. Under parliamentary privilege, he accused doctors at the hospital of 'carrying out lumbar punctures and a battery of other invasive tests on autistic children without proper research or clinical ethical approval'. He compared children studied at the Royal Free with 'research guinea pigs' and repeated his request for an independent public inquiry.

On the evening of 15 March, Harris stood before the House of Commons to set out his case in the most dramatic of terms. He charged that 'here is very clear evidence pointing towards unethical conduct by the [Royal Free] researchers – or by one or some of them – and equally strong evidence of failure and incompetence by the research ethics committee'. He quoted extensively from guidelines on research ethics published by the Department of Health in 1991 and the British Paediatric Association in 1992. He disagreed with the Royal Free's assertion that its research processes were 'subject to rigorous ethical analysis' of the sort and to the standard described in these official pronouncements. The incompetence shown by the hospital's ethics committee was 'shocking', he said. He demanded that the Department of Health 'investigate every ethics approval that the committee has ever given for research on children, to see whether anything else was allowed through – in effect, on the nod'.

These were merely his mild opening remarks. Harris then piled one extreme implication on top of another. He intimated, for example, that lumbar punctures might have been conducted 'as an excuse to obtain cerebrospinal fluid for private research contracts'. He suggested that 'doctors could face action for assault'. And he reflected on the possibility that, in addition to the GMC's inquiries, 'there may be another form of investigation – by the Crown Prosecution Service'. At the time of writing, as far as I know, not one of his allegations has been upheld and the investigations Harris has proposed have not been undertaken.

Harris's words did not produce any new evidence to throw additional light on the Wakefield research or the Royal Free's standards of ethics approval. Yet his comments were not so dissimilar in tone from the professional reaction not only to Wakefield's research but also to his outspoken claims at the Royal Free's press conference. Paediatric and public health experts were apoplectic over Wakefield's comments – and the *Lancet*'s decision to lend its credibility to his work. There seemed to be little room for calm reasoning. The *Lancet* report, and the legitimacy it gave to those who wanted to cast further (and unsubstantiated) doubt on the safety of the MMR vaccine, had to be opposed vehemently and absolutely.

Representatives from the Global Programme for Vaccines and Immunization at the World Health Organization, including its future Director-General, Dr Lee Jong-wook, called the publication of this paper 'tragic'.[8] We were told by others that we would 'bear a heavy responsibility for acting against the public health interest which you usually aim to promote'. A 'public health disaster' was predicted. The *Lancet* report 'provided a platform for the expression of views about MMR vaccination that have no proven scientific foundation'.

As the debate unfolded and became more refined in those early months of 1998, it was recognized by some critics that the finding of a potential link between autism and bowel disease was worthy of discussion.[9] This more balanced view was best summed up by Robert Chen and Frank DeStefano, who contributed a valuable commentary to put the original Wakefield paper into its proper health context. They noted that:

> We could not agree more that new potential adverse effects of medical interventions should be reported by clinicians as part of their Hippocratic responsibilities and rigorously scrutinized. However, the greater public good would be served if such 'signals' were reviewed through established safety monitoring systems designed specifically for this purpose . . . before claims of possible causality are promoted in medical journals or the mass media.[10]

Chen and DeStefano later went on to argue that the confusion surrounding the safety of the MMR vaccine indicated an urgent need for stronger vaccine safety monitoring systems, as well as better risk-communication strategies to maintain public confidence in vaccines.[11] This is the kind of constructive proposal that has so often been lost in the furious debate that followed Wakefield's report.

The professional uproar spread, of course, well beyond the pages of the *Lancet*. Careful reviews of laboratory-based studies concluded that there was no evidence of measles virus in bowel tissue of patients with inflammatory bowel disease.[12] Although these studies did not include children with autism, the research did successfully refute an earlier hypothesis, also put forward by Wakefield, that measles might in some way be a cause of these related bowel diseases. Since the MMR vaccine link to autistic enterocolitis sprang from these earlier claims, the demolition of this original foundation stone weakened considerably the logic, such as it was, underpinning the autism–MMR vaccine connection.

Elizabeth Miller was an especially acute critic of Wakefield and the *Lancet*.[13] As one of the leading vaccine specialists in the UK – she is head of the Immunization Division within the Health Protection Agency – Miller wrote scathingly of 'scare stories', 'astonishingly naïve' arguments, 'flawed statistics' and 'dubious' data. She concluded that our decision to publish Wakefield's work was 'a disservice to patients and health professionals alike'. Nevertheless, Miller was extremely careful not to dismiss Wakefield's claims without subjecting them to detailed critical analysis. Indeed, her style was quietly respectful to his arguments, despite her apparent anger. She conceded that his observations allowed 'clear and testable hypotheses to be formulated'. But when these hypotheses – for example, that the onset and incidence of autism were tied temporally to MMR vaccination – were tested, they were found to be wanting. She noted, rather ruefully, that: 'Clearly, to prove that the MMR vaccine could never cause autism is logically impossible because, indeed, to exclude the occurrence of a rare idiosyncratic association between any clinical event and a postulated causal agent would be impossible.'

But the fact was – and remains – that all of the evidence published to date, with the exception of that originating from Wakefield himself, offers no support to any claim of cause and effect between the MMR vaccine and a novel variant of autism. Miller herself became the subject of attack in March 2004.[14] *Private Eye* contrasted the perceived conflict of interest that we had levelled against Andrew Wakefield with those they claimed were held by Miller. The *Eye* argued that 'there is one rule for an off-message messenger like Dr Wakefield and quite another for the government and drug companies'. The magazine reported that Miller had been an expert witness for GlaxoSmithKline, Aventis Pasteur and Merck during the UK MMR vaccine litigation – a series of pharmaceutical and vaccine-manufacturer interests she had failed to declare in her published papers about the MMR vaccine. Indeed, in 2004 Merck was being accused of threatening families who believed that the MMR vaccine had damaged their children. The company suggested that parents might incur legal costs if they forced the vaccine manufacturer to defend itself. Was this a double standard for Miller? The *Eye* certainly thought so:

> Unlike the case of Dr Wakefield, there have been no screaming headlines attacking their credibility or honesty; no demands for an inquiry by the General Medical Council; no smirks at their 'fatally flawed' research . . . But every time [Dr Miller] now opens her mouth the question arises: Is she speaking from the 'impartial' view of the health department, open to all new research that comes to its attention; or for that of the defendant drug companies?

Miller replied that the *Eye*'s 'insinuation' suggesting she had 'become a mouthpiece for vaccine manufacturers is wholly incorrect'. 'I speak,' she wrote, 'from an independent scientific point of view within the interests of children's health.'

There is something wholly unsatisfactory about the way this debate has been conducted. It has been an anarchic free-for-all, coasting on the emotions of anxious parents, the publicity-seeking causes of a few opportunist politicians, the furies of public health officials, the despair of scientists and the glee of several newspaper editors. I am not advocating censorship of opinion. A plural public debate is vital. But the arrangements that we have in place to ensure just procedures for hearing all sides – Stuart Hampshire's central argument – and for testing the validity of evidence and opinion and for finding ways to resolve conflict are all patently failing.

Many of the elements needed to ensure rational public debate are already in place. We have, for example, a Chief Medical Officer within the Department of Health and a Chief Scientific Adviser within the Department of Trade and Industry, both of whom are respected and independent academic specialists, ideally placed to advise both the Government and the public. But the dispute over the MMR vaccine only shows the vulnerability of these government officials. When the controversy initially broke, the Department of Health made an unprecedented effort to provide the public with the best possible evidence about vaccine safety. In its 'MMR The Facts' campaign, the Department published letters, fact-sheets, frequently asked questions (with answers), information resource packs, leaflets, references, summaries of the myths and truths surrounding the MMR vaccine and supportive statements signed by the Royal College of General Practitioners, the British Medical Association, the Royal College of Nursing, the Faculty of Public Health Medicine, the UK Public Health Association, the Royal College of Midwives, the Community Practitioners and Health Visitors Association, the Royal Pharmaceutical Society, the Health Protection Agency and the Medicines Control Agency.

Dr David Salisbury, head of the Department of Health's section on immunization and infectious disease, together with Joanne Yarwood, the Department's head of immunization information, put enormous resources into attending eighteen parents' meetings and sixty-seven professionals' workshops in 2003 and 2004 alone. Their aim has been 'to share the information we have and to listen, understand, and address the concerns that people have'.[15]

Despite the energy of this campaign and the prestigious support offered for the MMR vaccine, many parents have remained unconvinced. The problem was well illustrated by the difficulty Sir David King, the Government's Chief Scientific Adviser, found himself in when he argued that the threat of climate change was greater than the threat of terrorism. He was immediately told to be silent by a government sensitive to criticism of its policies on terrorism, a controversial war in Iraq and its widely perceived genuflection before an aggressive US government.

The sad truth is that in the public's mind the British Government's scientific officials cannot easily maintain their reputations for independence. Even when the scientific information and advice coming out of government is accurate, the public not unreasonably asks if that advice is being manipulated for wider political objectives. Politicians have so damaged the civil service's reputation for independence that now even the advice of otherwise well thought of physicians and scientists within government is not entirely trusted.[16]

We face three crucial problems. First, we do not have the right language to discuss risk. Claims and counter-claims over risks are made and reported with equal vigour. Whether the chance of an event is quantified as one in 10 or one in 1,000,000, the mere fact that there is a risk – even a theoretical risk – seems to be enough to trigger public concern. To scientists, this seems deeply irrational behaviour. But thought of in any ordinary sense, it is profoundly rational. A risk implies an uncertainty, since the very meaning of the word 'risk' suggests an event that may strike at a place and time that are unknowable given our current understanding. Even if a risk is numerically tiny – say, one in 10 million – the fact that we do not know enough about that risk to be able to predict when exactly that one case will arise is sufficient to create a feeling of unease around any alleged risk-laden event.

Ken Calman was Chief Medical Officer at the time the Wakefield paper was published in 1998. He has written perceptively about the challenge of uncertainty in public conversations about risk.[17] Calman suggests several ways to improve our language of risk. We could seek to enhance public debate, although 'with fixed views on both sides, and with the intervention of the media, this process is unlikely to change minds'. A more formal process of public consent to a particular policy could be sought. But how? Through parliament? Or a national referendum? Perhaps dissent could be accommodated by allowing dissenters their preferred choice provided that there were no serious risks to others. Those who opted out of the mainstream would have to pay for their contrary choice and they would have to accept formally the consequences (and possible risks) of their decision.

The second problem we face is that we have very little knowledge about the way individuals, families and communities make decisions, such as those relating to whether or not to accept the MMR vaccine. We spend vast sums of money on research into new drugs, devices and vaccines – and almost none at all on what kinds of factors influence their use. The Department of Health argues that it does extensive consumer research about vaccines. But its officials also concede that very little of this work has been published. This dismal failure to communicate effectively reflects an entrenched complacency about public concerns surrounding vaccination. Instead, a common response from health professionals is to blame the media.[18] But this dismissal of the problem by blaming the messenger alone is a colossal misjudgement. In one series of focus groups about MMR immunization, for example, parents commonly described the 'unwelcome pressure' they felt from health-care workers.[19] Parents reported being bullied into accepting the vaccine. They were made to feel a nuisance if they asked questions. Government advice was 'insufficient to reassure parents about MMR's safety'. Parents sought a more open and less one-sided discussion with their doctor and they wanted more detailed information from independent and trusted (non-governmental) sources to help them decide on the best course of action for their child. As one group of investigators wrote, 'only by fully appreciating the concerns of parents will health professionals be able to work with them to restore their confidence in MMR immunization'.

This view has recently been strongly endorsed by a blue-ribbon panel of public health scientists put together by the UK's Wellcome Trust and led by Professor Stephen Frankel.[20] Their conclusions at last put the public at the centre of public health. Frankel's report is a profound criticism of a public health system that still reeks of nannying, paternalism and secrecy. In line with the spirit of Calman's analysis, Frankel's working group recommended that:

A more informed dialogue between public health scientists, the public, policy makers and the media must be engendered to develop a better understanding of risk in relation to health. This dialogue should be promoted through education, open presentations on the background to public policy and more collaborative engagement by public health scientists of the public, policy makers and the media. Policy and practice should be based on high-quality, empirical research, not on unevidenced assertions about the public's response.

The third and most important predicament facing the way in which society resolves scientific conflicts is the lack of any reliable institutional mechanism to allow differing points of view to be heard, discussed, challenged and, to the extent that they can be, resolved into a single consensus opinion. This is the lesson of Hampshire's *Justice is Conflict*. The controversy over the MMR vaccine shows the urgent need for such a mechanism. Wakefield informed the UK's Department of Health of his findings in 1997, and he subsequently sent the Department a final copy of the paper that was ultimately published in the *Lancet*. Just as Wakefield made ill-advised remarks at his now infamous press conference, so the Department of Health was unwise not to take Wakefield's claims more seriously in advance of publication. (Although the Department of Health claims that it did take Wakefield seriously going back as far as 1992.) And, I should quickly add, I too was ill-advised in not thinking through more carefully the way his group's findings might be misinterpreted at a press conference in the full glare of the media.

But as the *Times Higher Education Supplement* noted after the revelations of Wakefield's conflict of interest became public, 'for all the problems surrounding this research, unpopular opinions must still be heard'.[21] And yet no place exists where such unpopular opinions can be proposed and debated according to fair and accepted standards of evidence. The courts, for example, have failed all parents, irrespective of their views about the safety of the MMR vaccine. Litigation was irresponsibly supported by the Legal Aid Board, costing British taxpayers millions of wasted pounds. Hopes for a few families were unjustifiably raised, while the public scare over the vaccine was unreasonably sustained. The remaining institutions that we do have – Government, the Royal Society, the Academy of Medical Sciences, the Royal Colleges, the British

Medical Association – might once have all been suitable locations for open public dialogue. But that was in a more deferential age. That age has long gone.

When John Walker-Smith, one of the co-authors of the original 1998 *Lancet* paper, made his case for 'an independent research agenda' to study once and for all the alleged link between the MMR vaccine and bowel disease, where did he turn? When Simon Murch, also a co-author, declared that 'There is now unequivocal evidence that MMR is not a risk factor for autism', where did he go to make that assertion? When Peter Harvey, a third co-author, wrote of 'a step-by-step cascade of evidence . . . for a causative link between the MMR vaccine, a unique gastrointestinal disease, and regressive autism', where did he set out his evidence? The answer in all three conflicting cases was the *Lancet*.[22] While I would be one of the first to agree that a medical journal is a valuable forum to host debates of this sort, it is neither the best nor even the right place to arbitrate such contrasting opinions.

What Britain needs is a National Agency for Science and Health – NASH. Only an independent body such as NASH would provide the trustworthy space to debate and judge conflicting evidence concerning the health effects and ethical implications of mobile telephones, water fluoridation, genetically modified foods, animal experimentation, BSE and vCJD, SARS, stem-cell research, global warming, nuclear power, public health preparedness for weapons of mass destruction, organ transplants from animals to humans, gene therapy, the links between radon, cancer and housing design – and the safety of the MMR vaccine. NASH would be led by a prominent, scientifically literate public figure, but not necessarily by a scientist. It would draw on scientific expertise from existing national institutions and from international centres of excellence. Its multidisciplinary structure would include a strong thread of lay participation. There would be lay members on all its appointed committees of inquiry. These committees would have open evidence-gathering sessions, where the public and the media could attend and report on what they heard as the inquiry proceeded. Reports would be published. NASH would be sufficiently well funded to be able to commission its own research into public perceptions and attitudes to issues of concern.

The essence of NASH would be risk regulation. The agency would collect evidence about various potential risks, peer-review that evidence, quantify the risks as far as it could, and produce a list of priorities for public discussion. By acting prospectively instead of reactively, as government currently does, NASH would limit the damage caused by short-term flares of public concern, driven, as they often are, by marginal scientific opinions and a media hungry for controversy. NASH would be able to point out errors in popularly perceived risk estimates. One of its particular objectives would be to identify serious omissions in understanding so-called 'health–health trade-offs' – that is, the extent to which any proposed regulation implemented to diminish a health risk would actually introduce an additional new risk that was worse than the original one. NASH's work would involve regular systematic reviews of the evidence surrounding risks and their possible trade-offs, enabling it to constantly revise its risk estimates and judgements.

One of the methods that NASH would employ, therefore, would be a full accounting of risks and the effects of their proposed regulation – a kind of gain and loss account for any given risk. This accounting tool would demand the placing of all benefits of a given product or activity side-by-side with its potential harms. In the case of the MMR vaccine, this gain and loss approach would mean fully considering the risks of not having children vaccinated against measles, mumps and rubella infections versus the purely theoretical risk of the MMR vaccine causing a rare and anyway disputed complication.

A vital additional role for NASH would be the communication of its findings, as a means, if necessary, to correct public misperceptions about risk. The internet would be an especially valuable resource for providing risk information. NASH would offer an important and independent public information service, identifying the strengths and weaknesses of the arguments advanced and fought over in the media.

Too often, government relies on a command-and-control approach to public health. Ministers and public health officials issue mandates, proclamations and guidance with apparently little or no reference either to public attitudes about the activity being targeted (smoking, obesity, exercise and so on) or to an individual's capacity to respond to their injunctions. This deeply ingrained British political paternalism or 'nannying' – aided and abetted, unfortunately, by a public health leadership that is too often wedded to an unswerving belief in its own moral superiority – drives a damaging wedge between two communities that actually depend entirely on each other.

On the one hand, there is the public health community, which needs the support and confidence of a wider public if improvements to the health of the population are to be won. On the other hand, the wider public needs a vigorous public health system and a committed public health workforce if their own living and working environments are to become safer and healthier. The controversy over the MMR vaccine is just the latest health scare to put public and public health communities at odds with one another, and quite unnecessarily so. NASH would fill this trust deficit by providing a forum for deliberation and reflection over scientific evidence, public opinion and political choices. It would be free of any degrading commercial imperative. In this way, the new agency would play a substantial part in strengthening our democracy, in reviving civic rationality, in creating the space to resolve conflicts over evidence about risks, in countering pervasive and unjustified social fears, in providing the necessary and just procedural arrangements for doing so, and in answering questions about the nature of rational debate, some of which opened this chapter.

Of course, NASH does not exist at present. In preparing this book, I went to visit both Sir Liam Donaldson, the Chief Medical Officer, and Sir David King, the Government's Chief Scientific Adviser, to gauge their interest in the idea of a NASH.

Donaldson's office is in the Department of Health. A kindly official ushered me into a bare, faded-white waiting-room, reminiscent of general practice surgeries a generation ago. Orange rentacrates were stacked high on old wooden chairs. I felt myself becoming strangely nervous – a schoolboy about to be chastised by the stern headmaster. A few stony-faced office assistants passed by. A certificate noting that the Department of Health 'is recognized as meeting the national standard for effective investment in people (Jan 14, 1999)' hung in one especially gloomy corner.

It was 9.10 a.m. Donaldson was already running late and he seemed to be under pressure to be elsewhere. (The Minister had summoned him, he told me later.) The Chief Medical Officer has a disarmingly gentle bedside manner. He greeted me by clasping my hand in both of his, holding on to me for several seconds while delicately patting my hand as he did so. We sat alone on sofas opposite one another in his enormous office. A neatly dressed young woman brought us coffee poured into perfect bone china. Donaldson is as thoughtful and self-critical a person as one is ever likely to find in government. When I raised the subject of NASH, he was interested but not hopeful. He pointed to the Government's present drive to reduce bureaucracy. It was not a good moment to be proposing new institutions, he said.

Indeed, Health Secretary John Reid announced in May 2004 that there was 'considerable scope for improving efficiency and reducing bureaucracy' in health-service quangos. 'Arm's Length Bodies' (ALBs) sponsored by the Department of Health, such as the National Institute of Clinical Excellence, cost the nation £4.8 billion each year and employ 25,000 staff. Reid concluded that they encompassed many duplicated functions and that there was great scope for reducing or merging their activities. He wanted to shrink the number of ALBs by 50 per cent, save half a billion pounds each year, and cut 6,000 staff from the payroll. By July, he had announced his plans to do so.

King, whose Office of Science and Technology sits within the anonymous steel, glass, black leather and pine décor of the Department of Trade and Industry, was even more enthusiastic than Donaldson. He could envision some minimally bureaucratic linkage between existing national bodies. And he saw that the Food Standards Agency might be a useful model for NASH to measure itself against. But the reality was that the pressure to purge government of its quangos would be a likely brake on legislating to create any new independent agency.

There is a paradox here. I had originally written to Lord Sainsbury, the Parliamentary Under Secretary of State for Science and Innovation at the DTI. He politely passed me on to his Chief Scientific Adviser. The location of science within the DTI is telling. The foyer of the DTI on Victoria Street houses a large flat-screen television flashing the ministry's mission of 'prosperity for all'. Posters proclaim that the Department wishes 'to create the best environment for business success in the UK'. To do so, 'we invest heavily in world-class science and technology'. Science is therefore a means to a national end – the creation of wealth. The management of science must be about guarding and growing that wealth. Is there not a risk that science in the service of commerce will create an inevitable clash of values between corporate interests and public health concerns? Does this clash of cultures not require an independent, arm's-length means to mediate between them when certain issues become matters of supreme social torment?

If anyone still doubts the urgent need for the creation of a body such as NASH, they need look no further than the anguished and pleading testimonies of families caught up in the MMR vaccine controversy.[23] The mother of one boy who was reported to have been blinded and paralysed after contracting measles in 2003, following a reduction in his local community's herd immunity to measles, said, 'He [Wakefield] abused his power as a doctor by making the comments he did.' By contrast, some of the parents who believe that their children have been damaged by the vaccine wrote after Wakefield's paper was partly retracted:

We took our children to the Royal Free because they suffered from bowel symptoms (especially diarrhoea and pain) that no other centre was prepared to treat . . . There should now be a public inquiry into MMR safety. This shameful episode in modern medical science looks more like a Soviet show trial than scientific scholarship, as personal innuendo gives way to public accusations, retractions, and vilification. There is little thought for our children's future . . .

No civilized society can leave such conflicting views to hang so helplessly in the air. Yet still, nobody acts.

CHAPTER 3

The Dawn of McScience

'Virtue and morality, they say, cannot stand firm without the foundation of industry. Industry, by providing for daily necessities, and making life comfortable and secure for all classes of people will make virtue stable and common to all. This is all very well. Together with industry, at the same time low-mindedness, coldness, egoism, avarice, falsity, and treachery in commerce, all the qualities and passions which are most depraved and unworthy of civilized men, are in full vigour, and multiply endlessly. And we are still waiting for virtue.'

One unexpected benefit that followed from the partial retraction of Andrew Wakefield's research was the enormous public interest generated about financial conflicts of interest in science. The respected columnist Andreas Whittam Smith, for example, pointed out that conflicts of interest underpinned many of modern society's disputes and dilemmas, whether they took place in the courts, across government or among experts. Although conflicts of interest were sometimes hard to pin down, they did, he wrote, have a 'distinct pathology' that was observable in many different sectors of public life.[1]

George Monbiot enlarged on this theme in his characteristically outraged way in the *Guardian*.[2] Wakefield was, in Monbiot's view, only the tip of a very large iceberg. 'The scientific establishment is rotten from top to bottom, riddled with conflicts far graver than Dr Wakefield's,' he wrote. And, worse still, scientists too often fail to disclose them. Indeed, these 'daily deceptions' typify modern science. 'It's left to non-scientists to try to drag the data we need to see into the public domain.' He went on, warming to his argument, 'There is more corruption in our university faculties than there is in the building industry. But, though the mobs are baying for Wakefield's blood, hardly anyone in Britain seems to give a damn.'

The popular science press also raised a red flag. The magazine *New Scientist* argued that conflicts of interest 'fuel a perception that financial interests and competitive career pressures are so straining the integrity of research and the peer-review system that more policing is needed'.[3] The editors of *New Scientist* commented that 'nothing short of wholesale reform will do'. And, in particular, 'Perhaps the most profound conflict of interest in science today is that drug companies can choose which clinical findings they publish and which stay secret. Despite evidence that this practice can cause real harm, governments continue to allow it.'

But more specialist science publications were cautious in their assessment of these alleged problems. A degree of *realpolitik* was apparent in their editorial judgements, perhaps as a reaction to the wider press criticism of science and its collusion with the corporate sector. In an editorial entitled 'In no one's best interest',[4] *Nature*, Britain's most prestigious science journal, explained the reality of modern scientific research: 'Like it or not, we live in a world in which Mammon and science can walk hand-in-hand. Researchers often have a financial interest in the projects on which they work.' There was nothing inherently wrong about this state of affairs, the journal's editors argued. The solution – indeed, *Nature*'s editors presented it as a likely panacea – was disclosure. Provided everybody knew how connected an individual scientist was to a commercial interest, the problem would disappear. I believe that such an optimistic approach to the problem misses the important and irremediable compromise that science has had to make in its dealings with industry.

The view that *Nature*'s editors expressed after the Wakefield affair was best argued over a decade ago by Ken Rothman, a renowned epidemiologist from Boston, in what he called 'The new McCarthyism in science'.[5] Rothman not only questioned the importance of conflicts of interest, but also challenged the policy that many scientists and editors were then and now espousing – namely, disclosure as a measure to ameliorate the conflicts that will inevitably exist in all research.

Rothman claimed that the label of 'conflict of interest' was little more than a thinly disguised accusation of dishonesty. The idea that there was anybody in science – or in any walk of life, for that matter – who could attain a position of perfect objectivity was obviously wrong. Everybody, in one way or another, approaches a subject with a prior point of view. By focusing solely on financial conflicts of interest, the self-appointed guardians of science (he meant people like myself, the editors of journals) were undermining a long-held principle that work should be judged only on its merits. 'By emphasizing credentials,' Rothman wrote, 'these policies [of disclosure] foster an ad hominem approach to evaluating science.'

Disclosure of financial ties to a commercial sponsor suggests that the scientist has succumbed to some kind of poisonous bias. The mere presence of such a disclosure acts as a *caveat emptor* – an intellectual barrier between the reader and the work, indicating a health warning of sorts. The paranoia that was now prevalent in science concerning conflicts of interest had 'mushroomed into a policy of censorship'. Rothman wrote that '. . . these policies will reduce, rather than improve, the overall objectivity of scientific disclosure . . . the intent is to push readers and editors alike toward irrationalism . . . whenever we stray from using anything but the substance of a work itself as the basis for judgement, we begin to substitute prejudice for reason.' I can understand Rothman's argument very well. As soon as we pinpointed Wakefield's perceived conflict of interest as a key flaw in interpreting his claim that the MMR vaccine may be linked to autism, many other scientists, in a way reminiscent of the McCarthy-style method of imputing guilt by association, were paraded as being tainted by the brush of Mammon. The *Daily Mail* reported how nineteen government experts who sat on committees responsible for approving the safety of vaccines had 'interests' in the pharmaceutical companies that manufactured the MMR vaccine.[6] The charge against the scientific establishment was one of hypocrisy – and, to some degree anyway, it stuck.

Despite Rothman and despite calls in the immediate aftermath of Wakefield's disclosure for the *Lancet* to strengthen its conflict of interest regulations,[7] the fact was that we had already raised the profile of conflicts of interest substantially since 2001.[8] We not only now demanded disclosure of conflicts from scientists, peer-reviewers and even editors, but also we insisted that authors describe precisely the role of any funding source in the design of the study; the collection, analysis and interpretation of their data; the writing of the report; and the decision to submit the report for publication. These rules were and remain some of the strictest in operation at any journal today.

Are we over-reacting to concerns about the financial interests of scientists? Some critics may say so. But I prefer to trust the opinions of those people who take part in research – not the scientists and clinicians who do the investigations, but the patients who consent to take part in those studies. When potential research participants are asked whether it is important to know conflict of interest information – such as commercial funding, personal income, patent possession and stock ownership – most say that this information is, indeed, extremely or very important to know.[9] The strength of this feeling is even greater when they are asked whether this information should be made available as part of the process of informed consent. If public trust in the scientific enterprise is to be maintained, knowledge of conflicts of interest *must* be disclosed. But the issue is far more serious than the question of disclosure alone might suggest.

One of the most striking aspects of John Paul II's papal leadership has been his frequent and outspoken forays into science, especially the life sciences. His positions on abortion, sexuality and contraception have alienated vast numbers of Catholics and non-Catholics. Many people had seen his tenure in the Vatican as an opportunity for progressive leadership on issues ranging from AIDS in Africa to the reproductive rights of women. They have been disappointed. But his staunch orthodoxy has had one surprising, and some would say beneficial, consequence—a decisive opposition to the commercial exploitation of science.

In a letter to the apostolic nuncio in Poland on 25 March 2002, John Paul II condemned the 'overriding financial interests' that operate in biomedical and pharmaceutical research. These forces, he wrote, prompted 'decisions and products which are contrary to truly human values and to the demands of justice'. His particular target was 'the medicine of desires', by which he meant those drugs and procedures that are 'contrary to the moral good', serving as they do the pursuit of pleasure rather than the eradication of poverty. In an especially thoughtful passage, he wrote:

the pre-eminence of the profit motive in conducting scientific research ultimately means that science is deprived of its epistemological character, according to which its primary goal is discovery of the truth. The risk is that when research takes a utilitarian turn, its speculative dimension, which is the inner dynamic of man's intellectual journey, will be diminished or stifled.

Sheldon Krimsky, a physicist, philosopher, and policy analyst now at the Tufts University School of Medicine, puts it more bluntly. In *Science in the Private Interest*,[10] a strongly argued polemic against the commercial conditions in which scientific research currently operates, he shows how universities have become little more than instruments of wealth. This shift in the mission of academia, Krimsky claims, works against the public interest. Universities have sacrificed their larger social responsibilities to accommodate a new purpose—the privatization of knowledge—by engaging in multimillion-dollar contracts with industries that demand the rights to negotiate licences from any subsequent discovery.

Science has long been ripe for industrial colonization. The traditional norms of disinterested inquiry and free expression of opinion have been given up in order to harvest new and much-needed revenues. Universities have reinvented themselves as corporations. Scientists are coming to accept, and in many cases enjoy, their enhanced status as entrepreneurs. But these subtle yet insidious changes to the rules of engagement between science and commerce are causing incalculable injury to society, as well as to science.

This escalating corrosion of values derives from a sharp change in the political climate during the 1970s. The change first began in America. University administrators came to see their faculties as an undervalued resource. To counter what was viewed as a culture of financial passivity, the US Patent and Trademark Amendments (Bayh-Dole) Act of 1980 enabled universities to claim entitlement to inventions made with the support of federal funds. Suddenly university deans found themselves sitting on a mountain of unrealized income.

Scientists took to their new commercial calling with relish. Surveys reveal that a high proportion of researchers have ties to the industries whose products they are investigating.[11] Many have argued, and some no doubt believe, that money could never influence their scientific independence. But Krimsky makes a telling comparison with journalists and public officials, two groups for whom monetary conflicts of interest, now endemic in science, are anathema to their professional ethics. Instead, and this is surely a remarkable double standard, scientists absolve themselves from the dangers of often deep financial conflicts (such as company directorships, equity ownership, research grants, honoraria and travel costs) by the simple means of disclosure. Reporting a payment, a gift or other interest has indeed become a panacea, especially in medical journals, as *Nature* suggested in the aftermath of the latest round of Wakefield hysteria, allowing scientists to wash their hands of criticism.

This situation cannot be justified. Krimsky writes that 'the relationship between conflicts of interest and bias has been downplayed within the scientific community to protect the entrepreneurial ethos in academia'. But the damage inflicted by the influence of profit on the purpose of science has spread far beyond the university. The US federal advisory committees that dispense funds now give private interests priority over public ones. If committee members receive substantial payments from industries, this should in principle disqualify them from decisions affecting those industries. In the case of vaccine policy, for example, Krimsky quotes a 1999 US House of

Representatives Committee on Government Reform, which concluded that conflict of interest rules on Food and Drug Administration and Centres for Disease Control and Prevention advisory committees had 'been weak, enforcement has been lax, and committee members with substantial ties to pharmaceutical companies have been given waivers to participate in committee proceedings'.[12]

Even scientific journals, supposedly the neutral arbiters of quality by virtue of their process of critical peer-review, have their own difficult pressures to contend with. A piercing article by Shannon Brownlee in the April 2004 issue of the *Washington Monthly* underscored how perilous the position for medical journals has become. Brownlee simply put it this way: 'Why you can't trust medical journals any more.' She described how *Nature*, a partial advocate of conflict of interest disclosure in 2004, had only a few years earlier been caught out by the failure of one of its authors, in a closely related *Nature* publication, to declare an important conflict of interest. Only when a group of concerned doctors took their complaint to the *New York Times* did the story come to light. This episode reflected poorly on both science and one of its most highly regarded journals – but it also had implications for all editors. Brownlee quite reasonably asked: 'Why are the medical journals not more vigilant to weed out papers that have been distorted by conflict of interest?'

I know of editors who have been encouraged to adopt positions favouring industries that contribute substantial incomes to their journals, whether through advertising or from the sale of commercially valuable content. This is yet another example of the bias that has infiltrated academic exchange. As editor of the *Lancet* I too have attended medical conferences at which I have been urged to publish more favourable views of the pharmaceutical industry. For Krimsky, 'the idea that public risk (that is, publicly supported research) should be turned into private wealth is a perversion of the capitalist ethic'. The Pope would probably agree.

The idealism of Krimsky and the Pope – some would call it naïveté – could be a misleading guide in matters of scientific value. The notion that there was once some golden age of universal, communal, disinterested, and perfectly sceptical science, to use Robert Merton's famous tacit presuppositions about scientific cultures, is nonsense. Bertrand Russell was right when he argued that for as long as human beings have embarked on the activity we call science, their inquiries have had the twin functions of helping us to do as well as to know.[13] As Merton himself admitted, 'Readiness to accept the authority of science rests, to a considerable extent, upon its daily demonstration of power.'[14]

Yet this allegedly inescapable connection between science and technology has been challenged by a strain of historical study that finds a clear division between scientific inquiry and its more practical applications. For example, the American historian Steven Shapin, in his forceful exploration of the basis for scientific knowledge in the seventeenth century,[15] links the origins of English experimental philosophy with the cultural importance of truthfulness – 'the gentlemanly constitution of scientific truth', as Shapin puts it. He argues that our personal knowledge of the world depends to a large degree on what others tell us. Our understanding therefore has a moral character, based as it must be on trust. In constructing a body of reliable individual knowledge, trustworthy people are crucial. In the seventeenth century, the concept of the gentleman embodied these notions of trust. 'Honour' was the key to believing someone's testimony. Lying was seen as incompatible with a civilized society. A series of social conventions followed from this claim – the importance of face-to-face conversation, the centrality of 'epistemological decorum'.

In view of these conditions for truth, an opposition was bound to emerge between gentlemen and the trading classes. The merchant sought private advantages that created strong motives for lying. Deceit was pervasive in mercantile activities. Shapin quotes Erasmus: 'their lies, perjury, thefts, frauds, and deceptions are everywhere to be found.' And Robert Boyle, who discovered fundamental laws on the behaviour of gases, 'found by long and unwelcome experience, that very few tradesmen will, and can, give a man a clear and full account of their own practices; partly out of envy, partly out of want of skill to deliver a relation intelligibly'. Secret scientific knowledge and commercial exploitation of discoveries thus have a long and much-abhorred history within science, whatever scientists might claim in order to justify themselves today.

Still, most scientists and academic leaders will reject this negative attitude towards collaborations between science and industry. The argument for partnership seems entirely reasonable. Science aims to acquire knowledge, but needs money to invest in research. Industry wants to develop products for a profit, but needs a sound base of knowledge on which to do so. In other words, both activities need each other. Their interests are complementary. As the costs of basic science and clinical research have soared, thanks largely to the technological and organizational complexity of modern research, so universities have become more dependent than ever on the deep pockets of industry. The standard line advanced by corporate leaders is that these partnerships have been crucial to recent major advances in diagnosis and treatment of disease.[16]

But something changed dramatically in the early 1980s to push American academia and industry closer together. These forces were not accidental, and whatever today's rhetoric of complementarity and synergism might suggest, their consequences are not benign. The emerging biotechnology industry, based as it was on new techniques developed from molecular and gene biology, became the driving force behind this marriage of opportunities. The federal government enacted a list of statutes that mandated the National Institutes of Health (NIH) to cooperate with the private sector. Concerns were raised long ago by some academics about this changing landscape of science. Writing in 1991, William Raub, then acting director of the NIH, commented that,[17] 'the American body politic traditionally has erupted in anger when publicly financed activities yield undue private gain, when information intended for the many becomes the exclusive possession of the few, when personal goals are advanced at the expense of national ones, or when the prospect of profit breeds dishonest dealing'.

A decade later, many of these predictions have come true. When scientists ask colleagues to share their data, genetic discoveries, for example, are frequently withheld.[18] This proprietorial approach to new research findings is an increasing trend, especially in commercially sensitive disciplines. Lack of collaboration with other scientists prevents investigators from confirming and extending new discoveries. Contractual agreements between medical schools and industry sponsors of new research are also vulnerable in this culture of covert inquiry. The agreements fail to ensure that clinical trials follow widely accepted ethical practices, such as full protection of the patients enrolled in the study.[19] Contracts frequently contain no requirements for independent committees to monitor research and its safety. The access of an independent investigator to the trial's data is often not guaranteed. And usually there is no agreement that a trial's results will be published. These poor standards impugn the integrity of the entire field of biomedical research. And ultimately they put the well-being of patients at risk.

One case shows these difficulties all too clearly.[20] In the 1990s, Nancy Olivieri worked at the University of Toronto and at the city's

Hospital for Sick Children on a drug to treat a rare blood disorder called thalassaemia. Her work was sponsored by the Canadian Medical Research Council and a pharmaceutical company called Apotex. She discovered that the drug was not as effective as the company had originally hoped. Worse, the drug appeared to have very serious adverse effects. When Olivieri indicated her wish to publish her findings and inform the patients in her care of the drug's potential dangers, the company threatened her with legal action.

The hospital and university, which should have been the first to offer her protection from this outrageous intimidation, were the last to defend both her freedom to report her findings and her duty to act in the best interests of the patients under her care. Indeed, the hospital began an inquiry that failed to give Olivieri a fair hearing and other protections of due process. Astonishingly, she was fired. All this went on while the university was itself engaged in discussions with Apotex about a $12.7 million donation by the company to the University of Toronto. The president of the university was lobbying the Canadian government on behalf of Apotex.

After a further long and acrimonious investigation, Dr Olivieri was cleared of any alleged wrongdoing. Her reputation was restored and her position re-established. But the case ignited a furious debate within medicine about the moral responsibilities of investigators, their academic freedom, and the vital importance of strong institutional mechanisms to resist commercial forces that put stock value before professional ethics.

These institutional mechanisms are currently fragile. The purpose of the universities that support extensive research programmes is changing – inevitably and inexorably, say some of its leading analysts[21] – to meet an ever-greater need for money. More funds are necessary to secure top faculty, build new facilities and finance scholarships.

University administrators feel they have no choice: they have to move away from a mission based on the education of students to be informed and capable democratic citizens; instead, they have to concentrate more on producing people who can contribute to a 'knowledge economy'.

The problem is not only institutional. An extraordinary culture of gift-giving now exists within scientific research, a culture that has altered the way in which new discoveries are shared and debated. Take virtually any major medical conference. It is now entirely usual, among the many thousands of participants, for air fares, hotel costs, registration fees and evening entertainment (dinner, theatre, music) to be paid for by corporate sponsors, usually the pharmaceutical industry.[22] In return for this largesse, the conference organizers will hire space for an enormous trade exhibition at which the sponsors are allowed to display their products, services and promotional material, while offering even more gifts, such as bags, computer equipment, games, toys and clothes to its captive audience.

These meetings are usually billed as scientific gatherings. It is true that keynote lectures, together with research symposiums, make up a substantial proportion of the programme.[23] But the visitor cannot help being struck by the scandalous bargain that has been made between some professional societies and industry – namely that, in order for science to be reported and discussed among a professional society's membership, sponsors will be given the freedom to market their products to attending physicians. The venality of those taking part in this corrupt covenant is difficult to square with a profession that is quick to squeal at the mere suggestion of government intrusion into the delivery of health care. Any claim that the science and practice of medicine are disinterested is utterly groundless.[24]

About a quarter of scientists working in medical research have some sort of financial relationship with industry. And, not surprisingly, there is a strong association between commercial sponsorship and the conclusions scientists draw from their findings. Scientists who argue in favour of a particular product are more likely than their neutral or critical colleagues to possess a financial stake in the company that is funding their research or the product they are studying.[25] And, for the most part, these conflicts of interest are not reported when research is either presented at scientific meetings or published in medical journals. In my view, these findings are especially apposite when one considers the case of Andrew Wakefield and his funding by the Legal Aid Board.

Indeed, some medical journals have become an important but under-recognized obstacle to scientific truth-telling.[26] These journals have devolved into information-laundering operations for the pharmaceutical industry. Here is how it works. A pharmaceutical company will sponsor a scientific meeting. Speakers will be invited to talk about a product, and they will be paid a hefty fee (several thousand pounds) for doing so. They are chosen for their known views about a particular drug or because they have a reputation for being adaptable in attitude towards the needs of the company paying their fee. The meeting takes place and the speaker delivers a talk. A pharmaceutical communications company will record this lecture and convert it into an article for publication, usually as part of a collection of papers emanating from the symposium. This collection will be offered to a medical publisher for an amount that can run into hundreds of thousands of pounds.

The publisher will then seek a reputable journal to publish the papers based on the symposium, commonly as a supplement to the main journal. The peer-review process may be minimal or non-existent, and is sometimes not even the responsibility of the editor-in-chief of the parent journal. Publication of the supplement appears to benefit all parties. The sponsor obtains a publication whose content it has largely if not wholly influenced, but which now appears under the imprint of a journal that confers on the work a valuable credibility that the company has bought, not earned. The publisher receives a tidy high-margin revenue from the deal.

Why is this practice wrong and dangerous? The scientific quality of research in the thousands of industry-sponsored supplements published each year is notoriously inferior to the research published in properly peer-reviewed scientific journals.[27] The process of publication has been reduced to marketing dressed up as legitimate science. Pharmaceutical companies have found a way to circumvent the protective norms of peer-review. In all too many cases, they are able to seed the research literature with weak science that they can then use to promote their products to physicians.

Even what at first may seem like good research studies can hide far more sinister scenarios of buried bad news.[28] Clinical triallists, for example, can begin with the goal of studying one outcome, but, when that result is less favourable than the sponsor would have liked it to be, scientists may then choose (or be forced) to report an entirely different – and more positive – outcome. A team of Oxford University researchers, led by An-Wen Chan, concluded somewhat alarmingly that the results of clinical trials may be 'unreliable' and 'spurious', over-estimating the benefits of any particular treatment. Their findings represented 'the worst possible situation for patients, health-care professionals, and policy makers'. Some pharmaceutical companies go one step further. They may choose not to publish results that point to a lack of effect or problems with the safety of a drug. In 2004, GlaxoSmithKline was caught in one especially unpleasant storm over accusations that it had failed to publish research about an anti-depressant drug given to children and adolescents under eighteen years of age.[29] On the basis of these concerns, New York's attorney-general, Eliot Spitzer, filed a claim for fraud against the company. Under fierce criticism, GlaxoSmithKline disclosed results from multiple studies that cast their drug in a far more negative light than had hitherto been apparent through reading the available published reports.

Derek Bok, a former president of Harvard University, describes the damaging effects of this pervasive commercialization of science in his important report card on academia, *Universities in the Marketplace*. The concerns of research, he argues, have become skewed towards answering questions that are concerns of industry, not of the public. Secrecy disrupts a productive collegiality among scientists, leading to waste and inefficiency as investigators are forced to duplicate the hidden work of others. Opinions are rented out to the highest bidder. A nefarious web of incentives is introduced into research. And, most worrying of all, public confidence in medicine, science and the academy is undermined. Knowledge is just one more commodity to be traded.

The short-term effects of introducing a business culture into the academy may be so subtle that they will go unnoticed until it is too late to reverse their long-term consequences. Bit by bit, as Bok writes, 'commercialization threatens to change the character of the university in ways that limit its freedom, sap its effectiveness, and lower its standing in the society . . . The problems come so gradually and silently that their link to commercialization may not even be perceived. Like individuals who experiment with drugs, therefore, campus officials may believe that they can proceed without serious risk.' Is science, and especially biomedical science, now hopelessly compromised by its apparent dependence on industry?

Arnold Relman and Marcia Angell, both former editors of America's most respected medical journal, the *New England Journal of Medicine*, certainly think so.[30] In 2002, they wrote that the pharmaceutical industry, 'uses its great wealth and influence to ensure favourable government policies. It has also, with the acquiescence of a medical profession addicted to drug company largesse, assumed a role in directing medical treatment, clinical research, and physician education that is totally inappropriate for a profit-driven industry.'

The optimists who deny these arguments tend to fall into one of two camps. First, there is the growing view that science can be reclaimed for the public interest. Krimsky argues this case vigorously. For him, public interest science is 'research carried out primarily to advance the public good'. The values of public service in science need to be strengthened. Independent voices of dissent must be protected. The constraints on a scientist's freedom to think, write and investigate must be kept to a minimum. The business values of efficiency, assembly line production and the quest for utility need to be tamed.

How is this to be done? Krimsky and some other reformers believe that, whether in the academy or in the clinic, there should be a sharp separation between knowledge producers and wealth creators. All personal interests must be declared. If investigators have a direct financial stake – such as substantial stock ownership – in the outcome of research, they should not take part in it. And academic institutions with investments in particular corporations should not accept grants from those same companies.

An alternative view is that a dissolution of the partnership between science and commerce is neither possible nor desirable. Science is not merely about generating knowledge. It is about innovation. Businesses are increasingly 'outsourcing' their research and development costs – that is, they are allocating them to academic and other research institutions with which they make contracts. Universities have long had a valuable and justifiable part to play in fostering research into new medical remedies. Those scientists who wish to be entrepreneurs should be encouraged to develop an interest in their invention, not prevented from doing so, or so this argument goes. The crucial point is that rules should be put in place to ensure that these more commercially minded investigators are not permitted to conduct human research without tough independent oversight. In this way, the powerful incentives that drive scientific advance would be protected, while their more undesirable risks would be managed.

For such oversight to occur, however, universities, professional organizations, and scientific publications will have to improve many of their current practices and take a more demanding position towards private companies. It is far from clear either that this is what universities and professional organizations want to do or that there will be any effective sources of public pressure to make them change their ways.

The media is one useful means of applying necessary pressure for change. When the *Los Angeles Times* revealed in 2003 that senior scientists at America's leading research centre, the National Institutes of Health (NIH), were taking substantial consultancy payments from industry as well as a good government salary, politicians were angry. The director of the NIH, Elias Zerhouni, convened a blue ribbon panel on conflict of interest policies. Its draft report was leaked in April 2004, and the final report published a month later. The committee was chaired by the president of the US National Academy of Sciences, Bruce Alberts, and the retired chairman of Lockheed Martin, Norman Augustine. They considered that the NIH must exert stronger authority over the conflicts of interests of its employees. Its senior officials and those responsible for NIH grants should not accept paid consultancies with industry. Scientists should not be allowed to have financial interests in any company whose own interests may be affected by that individual's research. Any remaining financial relationships must be disclosed, the panel argued, not only in publications but also to patients as part of the process of informed consent. Some critics are still anxious that this new guidance does not go far enough to eliminate the influence of commerce from science. But if these recommendations are fully implemented, they would represent the most far-reaching overhaul of the links between business and academia for a generation.

Instead of possibly choking off innovation by legislating against the judicious commercial development of scientific research, a better way to proceed, according to John Ziman, a respected philosopher of science, is to let this work proceed unhindered while at the same time protecting the 'non-instrumental' functions of science that are currently under threat.[31] Ziman argues that the erosion of traditional scientific values – such as the principles that research should be driven by curiosity and by the desire to advance scientific knowledge – has created a new 'post-academic science', a science that seeks an immediate economic pay-off. Sustaining some form of non-instrumental science – which in practice means not routinely applying the litmus test of wealth creation to every new idea or hypothesis – is important not only for inquiry into fundamental theoretical questions but also because society needs a model of independent critical rationality for the proper conduct of democratic debate, judicial inquiry and consumer protection. But non-instrumental science can only be protected by organizations whose funding decisions are determined by disinterested scientists themselves, whether in university departments, charitable foundations or government agencies.

While Ziman's partial solution to the threat posed by private-interest science certainly sounds more practical than any desire to turn back the entire tide of commerce, it also poses its own dangers.

In a brief and tantalizing epilogue to his social history of truth, Steven Shapin speculates about the way trust and credibility are manipulated in the modern era. He notes that

> we are told things about the world [today] by people whom we do not know, working in places we have not been. Trust is no longer bestowed on familiar individuals; it is accorded to institutions and abstract capacities thought to reside in certain institutions . . . We trust the truth of specialized and esoteric scientific knowledge without knowing the scientists who are the authors of its claims . . . The gentleman has been replaced by the scientific expert, personal virtue by the possession of specialized knowledge, a calling by a job, a nexus of face-to-face intervention by faceless institutions, individual free action by institutional surveillance.

If personal virtue has indeed given way to impersonal expertise, and if moral character has become secondary to institutional prestige, it would be wrong to conclude that the connection between public trust and the integrity of the individual scientist has been wholly erased. But it has often become subject to a new set of institutional authorities. And this is a source of contemporary anxiety.

For if expertise is found to be shaped by motives of personal gain (as it increasingly is) and if the reputations of institutions are stained by private advantage (as they increasingly are), then trust will be as vulnerable to commercial corrosion now as it was to ungentlemanly behaviour in the salons of seventeenth-century English experimentalists. If these influences go unchecked, Thomas Hobbes's injunction 'against the lucrative vices of men of trade' could well become the dismal epitaph for modern science.

*

In Britain now, and despite the light shone on to conflicts of interest in science by the Wakefield affair, signs of relief from these pressures are not encouraging. In March 2004 the UK Government published a 'ten-year investment framework' for science called *Science and Innovation*. Noting that Britain led G8 nations in research productivity and that the UK has won more Nobel Prizes than any country except America, the Government's perspective was driven almost entirely by business considerations. The central challenge for science was that of maintaining 'future economic prosperity'. And the ambition for the Government was to achieve 'greater collaboration between universities and business to provide a sharper focus for research and an impetus to innovation and productivity growth'. The principle issues were those of 'commercial translation of leading edge technologies' and equipping 'the next generation of workers in the knowledge economy'. In particular, the Government sought better ways 'to maximize the benefits of investment from our partners in industry' in order to improve the 'economic rewards . . . in this crucial area of research'. Nowhere within the Government's strategy was there any recognition of the dangers posed by the excessive commercialization of science.[32]

What one can be certain of is that there will be increasing public debate about the over-zealous application of science in the private interest. There are likely to be many more examples of publication and research conduct that fail to meet the highest standards of probity. When these cases come to light, the press is the usual courtroom for these very public disputes. But the media cannot be the only place to charge, investigate, prosecute, defend, judge and pass verdicts on those who have been accused of impropriety, as we have seen.

In 2000, a group of UK medical journal editors, of which I was a member, drew attention to a collective institutional failure to take seriously allegations of research misconduct, of which conflicts of interest form a significant part.[33] The absence of formal mechanisms within many universities and at a national UK level to investigate claims with visible due process means that publicly aired allegations leave everybody involved scrambling to respond in the best way they can. Take the Wakefield affair. Once the claims and counter-claims about his actions were made public, multiple inquiries were demanded – into the way that ethics committees operate, into how the legal services commission makes its decisions, and, for the individual physicians concerned, by the General Medical Council.

This is no way to proceed. With no national body to which one can refer allegations such as those levelled against Wakefield and his colleagues, the danger is that in any ensuing media furore good people will be hurt by smear and innuendo. The appearance of institutions investigating themselves, while accepted as the current norm in science and medicine, does little or nothing to strengthen public trust in a system that has such critical societal influence, and thus which requires transparent lines of accountability.

Present scientific and medical institutions have failed to act after years of encouragement and embarrassment. It is now up to government to step in to create Britain's first Council for Research Integrity, modelled after similar bodies in Nordic countries.[34]

What would a Council for Research Integrity do? It would act as an independent oversight body, comprised of scientific and legal experts, an investigating branch, and a permanent administrative staff. Serious allegations of publication and research misconduct – such as the fabrication or falsification of data, disclosure of circumstances surrounding a piece of research that cast doubt on the validity of the findings, or issues of great public interest that had become clouded by accusations of questionable practices or ethics –

would be referred to the Council. A preliminary screen of these allegations by investigating staff would establish if there were grounds for further review. A committee of inquiry would then be established, made up of scientific and lay members and chaired by a person with legal training, to take evidence, hear all sides of the argument (Stuart Hampshire's 'audi alteram partem'), rule on the integrity of the research and its associated processes, judge whether the allegations were accurate or not, and finally make recommendations about how the parties should proceed.

The Council could also take on a broader role by establishing clear guidance on best scientific and research practice. This normative function could be its most important long-term contribution to science and society. It is difficult to think of reasons why a Council for Research Integrity should be resisted, other than the simple and understandable fear that the research enterprise would no longer offer the financial free-for-all that so enriches the few at the expense of the many.

I put the case for a Council for Research Integrity to Sir David King, the Government's Chief Scientific Adviser. While agreeing in principle that the problem needed to be tackled in some way, he was worried about creating a massive bureaucracy to crack what might prove to be a very small nut. This has been the concern of British scientists for a long time, and it is the main reason why the UK has failed to take the issue of research dishonesty seriously. But King was interested in the Scandinavian experience – an effective, minimally bureaucratic means to deal with allegations of misconduct. He seemed open to persuasion.

CHAPTER 4

Alone with Autism

'The most certain way to conceal the limits of one's own knowledge is not to go beyond them'

The National Autistic Society estimates that half a million families across the UK are affected by autism. A diagnosis usually comes after years of confusion and uncertainty. Two out of five children have to wait more than three years before an autistic spectrum disorder is confirmed. And once a diagnosis has been made, a child's subsequent experience can be fraught with difficulty. To take one very practical example – children with autism are twenty times more likely to be excluded from school than children without autism. The physical and emotional pressures on families affected by autism are huge and under-appreciated.

A great deal of the concern surrounding Andrew Wakefield's work has centred on parents with young children who are about to enter the age range at which the MMR vaccine is recommended. This anxiety is perfectly justified. Wakefield's specific advice to these parents was – and remains, I believe[1] – to consider seriously the option of single vaccines. Many friends of mine have sought out doctors who offer, at a considerable price, these individual vaccines. But as I discussed in Chapter 1, public health experts are rightly concerned that the provision of single vaccines would introduce genuine and far greater risks from natural infection with these three viruses – whose incidence would inevitably increase with a far less efficient vaccination regimen (six injections instead of two).

One group of parents is usually excluded from any public conversation in the media about the merits or otherwise of the MMR vaccine – namely, those with children who have been diagnosed as having an autistic spectrum disorder. They have become an even more marginalized group in the high-temperature debate over Wakefield's work. For parents who believe, for example, that the MMR vaccine is linked in some way to their child's condition, their testimony has been challenged and dismissed, sometimes cruelly I think, by those whose concerns lie with the wider public health protection of children against infection. The evidence quoted by these parents is described as 'anecdotal' and the value placed on their views by the original Royal Free physicians is rated as 'poor science'.[2]

Wakefield is correct to say that many of these parents have been poorly served by their doctors. He has written that 'their intestinal symptoms had been largely ignored'.[3] British medicine is extraordinarily good at providing care to those who need it immediately. In my experience, our acute medical services are second to none. But we are often extraordinarily bad – in terms of time, resources, and even expertise – when it comes to patients with complex and chronic conditions. Autism is one such condition, and especially so for the variant of autism described by the original Royal Free team, which seemed to defy all known understanding of the disorder.

What has been the effect of Wakefield's work on these parents? And what implications are there for those charged with advancing our understanding of this mysterious condition?

One place to look for an answer to the first question is the enormous stack of self-help books now available for parents of children with autism. Simply by combing the shelves of well-known bookstore chains in early 2004, I could find well over a dozen such books. A close reading of their authors' interpretations of Wakefield's work gives cause for alarm about the way health research is read, digested, applied and disseminated by writers and publishers. And I should add here, too, that the imprint of Wakefield's views on this literature gave me even greater reason to worry about the way our original decision to publish his findings had been used to lend authority to claims that were not only wholly unjustified (that the MMR vaccine was a cause of autism) but also completely absent from the original paper.

I found thirteen books that discussed Wakefield's work.[4] Four were either by parents of children with autism or by journalists with an interest in autism. Nine were by academics, health professionals who work with children who have autism, or writers who claimed to be producing balanced accounts for parents. Although there was a sharp division between the two groups in the way that they looked at Wakefield's findings, there were signs of endorsement for Wakefield's extreme position on the safety of the MMR vaccine from sources that I would have expected to present a more critical appraisal of his work.

But let me turn to the parent–writers first. The value for any parent with a child who has autism of reading a book by a fellow parent is particularly high. A parent is almost bound to feel that they are getting the unvarnished truth about a condition, free of cold, impersonal technical jargon and the overly medical or biological approach that is thought to be commonly provided by doctors. Parents are more likely to disclose to one another the hidden facts about how to cope with such an unwanted diagnosis. They will offer shortcuts to understanding the reality and meaning of their child's condition. They will help fellow parents avoid the common pitfalls that are likely to befall them. They will provide a sense of a community for families that are going through the same trying set of experiences. No parent, these books correctly proclaim, needs to be alone with autism. And yet when it comes to Andrew Wakefield and his views on vaccines, these books almost always disappoint.

Lynn Hamilton is 'a speaker who shares her family's experiences with autism'. In *Facing Autism*, she offers ten pieces of advice to help parents. Number nine is 'Postpone Vaccinations'. She writes:

> Recent findings in the medical world have caused many parents and physicians to take a second look at vaccines . . . What I stress here is that you consider postponing any vaccination for your child with autism *and* your other children until you have time to research more information and perform any relevant tests. I'm not suggesting you withhold vaccines forever, but I do urge you to wait until you're able to make an informed decision for each of your children.

Hamilton begins two of her chapters with quotations from Wakefield, whose views she seems to endorse.[5] Hamilton reports that he has called 'for the cessation of the MMR combination vaccine'. She asks, 'Intellectually, we understand that vaccines will never be 100 per cent safe, but what if our children are among the few injured by the vaccine? . . . Could autism be connected to vaccines?' And she answers that question by describing how she has decided not to give her own son, who has autism, a second dose of the MMR vaccine. Hamilton advises parents that they may feel pressured to accept the vaccine. She urges, 'Don't be intimidated, this is your child and your decision. Take time to choose wisely.' She concludes by inviting parents to think about using single vaccines 'to avoid overloading the child's immune system'.

Stephanie Marohn is a medical journalist. In her book, *The Natural Medicine Guide to Autism*, she acknowledges that Wakefield's work has generated 'huge controversy'. But she does not flinch from giving advice for potentially confused families:

In reviewing the literature, it seems evident that there is at least reasonable doubt regarding the safety of certain vaccines. Why then are they not pulled off the market while further study is undertaken? When you consider the stakes involved, the answer becomes clear – and it has a dollar sign in front of it . . . The MMR vaccine seems to be particularly problematic for children who are susceptible to developing autism . . . Dr Wakefield's conclusions are supported by other medical professionals and researchers . . . Many people who have researched the subject believe that the number of different viruses given at one time is part of the reason for the great increase in autism.

Marohn frames her interpretation of the scientific evidence within the context of an individual – Andrew Wakefield – who has become 'the target of virulent criticism and attack'. The 'attempts to discredit' him are 'amazing', she writes, given 'the measured, scholarly content and careful conclusions' of his work.

Patricia Stacey is a writer whose son has autism. In *The Boy Who Loved Windows*, she tries to present the debate about the MMR vaccine in a more balanced way, but in doing so gives undue credibility to a set of opinions largely refuted by the overwhelming majority of experts who have studied the evidence. She uses colourful language in her portrayal of Wakefield's concerns: '. . . since the advent of vaccinations, the kind of autism that appears at eighteen months, once considered rare, began appearing with shocking frequency as these changes in vaccination patterns occurred.' To be fair, she does point out that critics claim Wakefield's work is 'flawed'. But her style – on the one hand this piece of evidence, on the other hand that piece of evidence – gives the false impression of a perfectly even scientific debate, which is simply incorrect.

Adelle Tilton is also the parent of a son with autism. She has written a book the title of which claims to be *The Everything Parent's Guide to Children with Autism*. She describes vaccination as 'one of the leading theories behind the cause of autism', and the MMR vaccine specifically as a 'leading subject'. Once again, she reports the evidence in a way that clearly displays her own view about the safety and value of the trivalent vaccine:

> Some leading studies have shown that upon biopsy of the lower gastrointestinal tract of children with autism, measles is found. This, of course, is not normal, and since many children with autism also have bowel diseases, it raises the question of what the connection may be . . . The research continues, and in the interim, many parents have decided against immunizations, despite the insistence of health organizations that there is no link between the MMR [vaccine] and autism. There are thousands of anecdotal stories about children who were perfectly normal until shortly after the first MMR immunization. These children spoke in phrases, interacted with people around them, and suddenly became nonverbal and non-responsive within a few days of receiving the immunization.

I found all four of these parent-to-parent guides to be profoundly disturbing. Why was the case *for* vaccination not made? Why was the burden of illness and disease caused by measles, mumps and rubella infection not explained? Why were the many epidemiological and laboratory studies contradicting the claims of harm attributed to the MMR vaccine not described? Why was the available evidence treated in such an even-handed way when, in truth, it is highly skewed towards those who attest to the vaccine's safety? Why had the authors failed to provide the best available medical advice to their readers? Why had their editors and publishers allowed them to do so?

The remaining nine books by health writers or health professionals working in the fields of medicine or education present more sceptical views of Wakefield's work. The best parental guidebook on offer is by Lorna Wing, a respected academic psychiatrist who has made substantial contributions to our understanding of autism throughout a long career. She is also the mother of a daughter with autism.

In *The Autistic Spectrum*, Wing acknowledges that there has been 'great concern' that the MMR vaccine might cause autism. In judging the 'weight of the evidence', she concludes that 'there is no solid evidence for this theory'. She goes on to explain the then (2001) state of understanding in what I think is a model of how to present complex scientific evidence to a wider public audience – that is, respecting the intelligence of readers by giving detail, but at the same time giving clear guidance about the credibility of that evidence:

> One team of research workers has reported finding abnormalities of the lymphoid tissue, containing the measles virus, in the lining of the intestines in children whose parents believe that autism began after MMR vaccination. They attribute the feeding and bowel problems to this. Their findings have not, so far, been confirmed by other investigators.

By contrast, Bryna Siegel, an autism expert who directs a clinic at the University of California, San Francisco, is, in my view, too dismissive, failing to address the likely concerns of families: 'Sometimes autism is blamed on things that are common, like infant vaccinations . . . this is about as logical as saying that autism is caused by drinking orange juice.' The respected neuroscientist Uta Frith describes the MMR vaccine as a 'scapegoat' and its suggested link to autism as an urban myth. Parents' perceptions are simply 'fallible'.

Diane Yapko, a Californian speech-language pathologist, dithers. She argues that 'research to date does not support a direct link between the MMR vaccine and autism', but she argues that 'the observations and common experiences reported by physicians and families keep the research alive'. She writes of the vaccine as 'a possible cause of autism'. Fiona Marshall, a medical writer, concludes that 'the consensus seems to be that the majority of medical evidence is against vaccines causing autism, though there may be a possibility that the vaccine contributes to the disorder in a small number of vulnerable children'. Chantal Sicile-Kim discusses the uncertainty surrounding the vaccine but notes that 'what is real is the growing number of parents who have seen differences in their children before and after the MMR vaccine, and have photographs and videos that clearly document regression. This is a fact for those families that no government report will erase.' And Marlene Targ Brill urges parents to 'weigh the pros and cons' of vaccination, after reporting that 'the rise in autism worldwide has mirrored an increase in vaccinations as directed by World Health Organization policy'.

And two writers, both American – one a professor of special education, the other a specialist in environmental medicine – make many of the same errors as the non-specialist authors I have quoted. But their professional credentials lend unjustified weight to concerns about the safety of the MMR vaccine. Shirley Cohen, an educationalist, reports Wakefield's view and asks,

> Why are multiple vaccines routinely administered to infants on the same day? Why aren't the components of the MMR vaccine available separately? . . . The role, if any, that the current heavy schedule of vaccines administered to young children plays in the increasing number of children identified as having autistic spectrum disorders is an issue in serious need of further study.

Meanwhile, Stephen Edelson, while accepting that Wakefield's theory has 'been almost totally discredited', concludes on the basis of no evidence that vaccines 'may in some cases trigger or push over the edge a case where a child's immune system is already compromised'. Many of these writers give a one-sided view of present scientific understanding about the autism–bowel–disease–MMR–vaccine hypothesis. Taken together, they have contributed to the manufacture of fear surrounding the MMR vaccine, a fear that has proven impossible to alleviate.

The story of autism is one that should make all doctors and parents alike pause before they pronounce with certainty on the origins of a disease. In the official history of medicine, the phenomenon of autism began with a paper published by an American psychiatrist, Leo Kanner, in 1943.[6] He described eleven children with a condition that differed 'markedly and uniquely from anything reported so far'. He believed that the characteristics of these children, the fundamental feature of whom was their 'inability to relate themselves in the ordinary way to people and situations from the beginning of life', constituted a syndrome, one that he described as 'an extreme autistic aloneness'. The recognition of such a distinct clinical entity was important, even urgent at that time. Kanner described how several of the children who had been introduced to him were inappropriately labelled as 'idiots or imbeciles'. One lived in a 'state school for the feebleminded, and two had been previously considered as schizophrenic'.

At the close of his remarkable article, Kanner indulged in what now seems rather distasteful speculation. Although he concludes that autism is innate, he also pointed out that there was an unusual degree of 'parental obsessiveness' in the families he had evaluated. In particular, there were 'very few really warm hearted fathers and mothers'. The marriages that he observed, when they had not been 'dismal failures', were 'rather cold and formal affairs'. Here was the beginning of an era distinguished by professionals who laid the blame for autism directly on the shoulders of parents.

The apotheosis of this approach came with the work of Bruno Bettelheim (1903–90). Born in Vienna and imprisoned in Dachau and Buchenwald from 1938–9, Bettelheim thereafter moved to the US, where he applied theories of psychoanalysis to children with autism.[7] He believed, not unfairly, that the most extreme agony a child can feel is to be utterly forsaken. But in autism, Bettelheim saw children as the victims of icebox mothering. According to Bernard Rimland, a noted expert on autism, Bettelheim 'proclaimed that autistic children had been mistreated by their mothers in about the same way in which Nazi concentration camp prisoners had been mistreated by their guards, thus giving the children (like the prisoners) feelings of hopelessness, despair, and apathy, and leading them to withdraw from contact with reality'.[8]

Bettelheim's style today does seem imbued with a perverse insensitivity. In a celebrated article published in *Scientific American* in 1959, he described the story of 'Joey: A "Mechanical' Boy". Joey, Bettelheim claimed, 'presented a classic example of . . . infantile autism'. But he was a child who, first and foremost, 'had been robbed of his humanity'. Bettelheim did not hesitate to blame Joey's parents, especially his mother, who was almost entirely 'preoccupied with herself'. She was 'fey', insecure, detached, lacked vitality, and seemed totally indifferent to her son. Joey was treated like a machine: 'As a toilet-trained child he saved his mother labour, just as household machines saved her labour. As a machine he was not loved for his performance, nor could he love himself.'

Not surprisingly, many parents with children diagnosed as being autistic reacted angrily to claims that the origins of their child's illness lay in the home. Parent-support organizations sprang up to represent the interests of these aggrieved families. For example, in the UK, the National Autistic Society was launched by parents in 1962 to encourage greater understanding of the condition. The Society now has over 12,000 members, national and regional councillors, a board of trustees, a senior management team and a chief executive. The actress and writer Jane Asher is its President and the Countess of Wessex its Royal Patron.

Questions about issues such as the safety of the MMR vaccine put the National Autistic Society in a very difficult position. As an organization created by and for parents of children with autism, there must be a natural tendency to cleave towards the views of parents, some of whom passionately believe, against the opinions of the medical establishment, that the vaccine is the cause of their child's condition. The fight initiated by these parents must seem reminiscent of the struggle forty years before against the received professional wisdom of the time. And yet as a registered charity and as the official voice of the autism community in the UK, the credibility of the Society very largely depends on maintaining strong alliances with politicians – through the All Party Parliamentary Group on Autism – and the medical community. One can sense this tension in the Society's published position on the safety of the MMR vaccine. In one statement, for example, the Society acknowledges that 'the general medical consensus at present is in favour of vaccination and we accept that in most cases the benefits will far outweigh the costs'. This conclusion in favour of the vaccine seems almost grudging – notice, for example, the phrase 'in most cases'. The Society's solution to this difficulty is to call for more research, arguing that our present understanding about the role of vaccines in causing autism is 'inconclusive'. In a separate statement issued in July 2003, the Society avoids adopting a position in a way that seems to contradict one of its very reasons for existing. The Society declares that it 'Cannot, and does not, advise parents as to their best course of action . . . it is unable, therefore, to state whether or not there is any link between any vaccine and autism.'

Thanks to the work of campaigners such as Rimland, scientists such as Michael Rutter, and parents such as those who created the National Autistic Society, psychological theories of autism eventually gave way to more biological explanations.[9] The origins of autism almost certainly lie in the developing central nervous system: anatomical abnormalities in various parts of the brain have been identified, including disorders of brain growth; changes in brain chemistry have been described; and seizures are more common in children with autism.

The major present focus of interest, like in so many other areas of medicine, is genes. New genetic associations and disorders potentially linked to autism are regularly reported in medical journals. In any survey of recent research publications on autism, over a quarter are devoted to studies of genes – the MMR vaccine comes a distant second. In April 2004, *The Times* (rather hyperbolically) announced that 'scientists identify a first gene for autism'.[10] A team of investigators from New York had found that a gene on chromosome 2 increased the risk of developing autism at least two-fold. In truth, this gene is likely to be one of many that influence the chances of developing this condition. Different genes may be involved in different variants of the disorder and at different times in the development of the brain.

The innate nature of autism has also led to great efforts to design methods to detect early symptoms of the condition. The value of an early diagnosis mainly lies in the provision of quick access to care services. Families prefer to know a diagnosis sooner rather than later, especially when later can mean a painful course of wrong diagnoses and multiple referrals to puzzled specialists. A further advantage of early diagnosis is that the chance of having a second child with autism is about one in twenty – ten times the usual rate of occurrence. This information may be helpful for parents who are deciding whether to extend their family.[11]

But there is another side to the origins of autism, one that is relevant to the story of how the MMR vaccine came to be entangled with this condition. In 1989, the distinguished autism investigators Fred Volkmar and Donald Cohen described a late-onset type of the disorder.[12] They reported children who experienced an interval of normal development followed by the beginning of rapid regression or 'disintegration'. The creation of this new but rare diagnostic category raised the possibility of some kind of triggering event that underlied the regression. No trigger has yet been identified, although obviously the MMR vaccine has been suggested as one such precipitating cause.

There is an intriguing history to be reflected on here. For example, in 1978 Stella Chess and her colleagues described an unusually high rate of autism following an outbreak of rubella infection.[13] Of 243 children with congenital rubella, eighteen were diagnosed as having classic Kanner-type autism (7.4 per cent). At that time, the expected frequency of autism was 0.7 per 10,000. The rate reported by Chess was 1,000 times higher. To add a further twist of interest to this line of investigation, an American research group detected season-of-birth effects for particular groups of children with autism. In one collection of children from Boston, there was a peak frequency of births of children with autism in March. Michael Stevens and his colleagues concluded that they might have discovered evidence for an 'environmentally related autistic disorder'.[14]

The truth is that scientists have a very poor understanding of what the environmental triggers for autism might be. It seems clear that events taking place during pregnancy and around the time of birth are important influences. But what might these influences be? The research to date is crude and unhelpful, at least for parents worried about whether their child is or is not susceptible to autism. As I scan the many studies that have been completed, I can find references to maternal age older than 35 years, fetal distress, fetal growth difficulties, caesarean section, epidural anaesthesia, induction of birth and a short duration of labour. This collection of risks makes no coherent sense. It is even alarmist. A caesarean section is not a 'cause' of autism. A caesarean section is probably a proxy risk factor that hides other, most likely unknown, phenomena affecting the chances of a child developing autism. To add to this complexity, scientists have no idea how these risks are altered by the presence or absence of particular genes. Any reasonable person approaching the subject of autism for the first time would be astonished at how little modern medicine has discovered about this extremely common condition.

Yet there are dangers of careless reductionism in this now expanding strain of biological research. Just as psychological theories led to blame being placed on parents, so more organic explanations can turn children into objects. Consider this discussion of those who live with autism by the celebrated psychologist, Steven Pinker:[15] 'Together with robots and chimpanzees, people with autism remind us that cultural learning is possible only because neurologically normal people have innate equipment to accomplish it.'

Although our understanding of autism has progressed considerably beyond the simplistic metaphors and questionable motivations of Bruno Bettelheim, this kind of equation (child with autism = robot = animal) reminds us that the tendency to strip away the humanity of children with autism has not been entirely erased from science.

Part of the difficulty in understanding autism is that we have a very poor conception of what autism actually is. I used to work in Birmingham and London with patients who had liver disease. These patients were frequently jaundiced. Their yellowed skin was an outward sign that they had liver disease. But the fact of being jaundiced told me little about what was actually going wrong inside that person's body. To understand the external sign of jaundice, I needed to have a set of concepts explaining what the liver is and what it does. I needed to understand its anatomy, its three-dimensional structure, how that structure related to the organ's normal function, and what happened when that normal function was disturbed or interrupted by disease.

The same is true – or would be true if only we knew more – about autism. Autism is a condition that is now known to have a wide spectrum of behaviours – hence the more commonly used term 'autistic spectrum disorders'. At its most fundamental level, autism encompasses impairments in normal social skills, disturbances in speech, language and communication, an absence of imagination, the need for predictability and routine, over-attention to some stimuli in the environment (e.g., certain sounds) and under-attention to others, and a different pattern of early development, especially in social interaction.

Children with autism also display unusual repetitive behaviours, such as rocking back and forth while standing, hand- and arm-flapping, and jumping. But these surface characteristics of autism, like the jaundice of liver disease, tell us very little about the underlying nature of the condition. And without understanding the neural mechanisms behind autistic behaviours it is hard to design appropriate treatments. One difficulty is that, beyond a simple list of common symptoms and signs, doctors do not have a clear and specific concept of what autism is.

Some of the most illuminating – and certainly the most intriguing – work into the fundamental basis of autism comes from Simon Baron-Cohen, a British psychologist who, together with many colleagues, in particular Uta Frith, has developed a coherent, compelling, and testable theory of autism – in fact, a theory of mind of children living with autism.

What is a theory of mind? Each of us is usually able to conceive the idea of mental states. We understand that other human beings have mental representations of the world. It is not hard for us to accept that other people can think, feel and believe. We are able to draw conclusions about the way in which others might think about a particular situation. For example, if I see you getting into the driver's seat of a car, I may reasonably infer that you are about to start the car and drive away. This ability to predict what you might do by trying to conceive your mental state at the moment you get into the car is called a theory of mind.

In a now classic article published in 1985, Baron-Cohen, together with his colleagues Uta Frith and Alan Leslie, asked whether the child with autism has a theory of mind.[16] After

106

conducting a simple but elegant experiment in a small group of children, they concluded that many children with autism lack a theory of mind. These children were unable to accurately predict behaviour by imputing beliefs to others. Further work has indicated that although a small proportion of children with autism do have a theory of mind, it is very delayed in its appearance.[17] Not only was a theory of mind absent or delayed, but also, when it did emerge, its components – an appreciation of perception, desire, imagination, pretence and belief – developed in a different sequence compared with children who did not have autism.[18] There are now the beginnings of attempts to correlate theory of mind impairment to brain function[19] – the first step in developing a true conceptual picture of autism.

Baron-Cohen has called the absence of a theory of mind in children with autism 'mindblindness'.[20] It is not the only theory of autism under discussion among experts, but it is certainly one of the more intriguing ideas around. Baron-Cohen has, for example, more recently moved his theory of autism on to territory almost as controversial as that occupied by Andrew Wakefield – namely, that of the supposed innate psychological differences between men and women.

In a highly provocative and engaging book, *The Essential Difference*,[21] Baron-Cohen argues that 'The female brain is predominantly hardwired for empathy. The male brain is predominantly hardwired for understanding and building systems.' And here is where autism fits in. Baron-Cohen argues that 'Autism is an empathy disorder.' People with autism find it hard or even impossible to put themselves into a position where they imagine themselves to be in somebody else's mind. He quotes Hans Asperger, who described a syndrome that is now part of the autistic spectrum. In 1944, Asperger wrote that 'The autistic personality is an extreme variant of male intelligence,' a view that Baron-Cohen endorses by calling autism an example of 'the extreme male brain'. The child with autism is different, not disabled. Difficult questions remain unanswered, of course. Why does a theory of mind fail to develop in these children? And would developing a theory of mind help to ameliorate the problems that can cause so much discomfort to the children who live with autism?

These questions have become urgent because of the changing nature of 'autism' in recent years. A decade ago, the prevalence of autism – as defined by Kanner's original criteria – was roughly five children out of every 10,000. It was the rarity and yet the severity of the condition that led writers such as Lorna Wing to note that these children's difficulties were 'often intensified by lack of recognition, even denial that autism exists, among some medical and other professional workers'.[22] But the prevalence of autism is now sometimes reported to be as high as one in 200 children – an explosion, some might even say an epidemic, of cases.

These dramatic changes in frequency are hard to explain. And the way that this uncertainty is portrayed to the public creates fertile ground for new theories about autism's causes, irrespective of whether they have the confidence or not of most experts. Take, for example, a front-page report in the *New York Times* on 26 January 2004. The headline read: 'Autism cases up; cause is unclear.' A smaller headline beneath that opening declaration explained: 'Some see an epidemic – others express doubt.' Erica Goode, one of the newspaper's top medical journalists, began her article by noting that cases of autism were indeed 'rising sharply', a fact that 'no one disputes'. She cited figures showing that cases had tripled from 1987 to 1998, and then doubled from 1998 to 2002 – alarming by any standards.

But why the sudden change? Goode quoted experts who simply

put it down to increased public and professional awareness of this 'baffling and often devastating neurological disorder'. Others believed that something more sinister was happening, that we were truly all caught in the middle of an autism epidemic. It was vital to find an answer either way, because only then would scientists know with how much vigour they should be 'tracking down environmental factors in addition to genetic influences'. This is the very uncertainty, of course, that those predisposed to Wakefield's claims pounce upon.

Goode pointed out that some patient advocacy groups have talked of a public health crisis regarding autism. They argue that a real increase in cases of the disease must prove the existence of a new environmental trigger. Goode quotes several candidates – infections, thalidomide, plastics and food additives. And, of course, the MMR vaccine. Although she dismissed the evidence for all of these supposed 'causes' of autism, her article left the strong impression that at least some of the increase in autism's frequency was due to genuine rises in prevalence and not merely better diagnosis. The question was how much of the increase. The more that one believes the increase is genuine, the more urgently one will want scientists to be searching for some so-far unknown precipitating cause. The more one believes the increase is a result of better awareness, the more one will think that we should simply concentrate on working harder to improve care and education services for those who are affected.

Yet my survey of the available evidence in 2004 indicates a far clearer picture than this article suggests. If one examines the published, peer-reviewed research on the prevalence of autism, it seems to me that experts believe we are dealing with higher awareness and improved diagnosis[23] – an important but otherwise benign phenomenon.

This is a view that is also shared by the man who first identified a late-onset variant of autism, Fred Volkmar, as well as by the indefatigable Lorna Wing. Rates of autism have risen from about four per 10,000 children in the 1970s to fifty or sixty per 10,000 children today. In one study completed in Cambridgeshire, Fiona Scott, Simon Baron-Cohen, and their colleagues at the University of Cambridge looked at children with autism spectrum disorders aged between five and eleven years of age. They found 196 children with a confirmed autism spectrum disorder – a prevalence of fifty-seven in 10,000 children, over ten times the expected rate.

Wing considers seven explanations for why these frequencies have risen so steeply. The first is that there has simply been a change in the diagnostic criteria for autism, thereby widening the net for detecting children with milder forms of the disorder. This reason will likely explain some although not all of the increase. A second possibility, which is hard to rule out, is that the differences are spurious, reflecting only differences in the way individual studies have been conducted and reported – the harder one looks, the more autism one finds, for example. It is difficult to imagine that this arte-factual cause, based as it must be on scientific inconsistencies and errors, lies behind the commonly reported increases in frequency seen in recent years.

A much more important third reason may be an increased awareness of autism among families and health workers. The creation of parents' organizations, such as the National Autistic Society, has raised the visibility of these conditions among the public and politicians alike. Among scientists too, autism has become a legitimate and serious area for research. (And a subject for curiosities too. In 2004, two psychiatrists, Muhammad Arshad and Michael Fitzgerald, proposed that Michelangelo might have suffered from a high-functioning type of autism, thereby explaining his obsessive work routine, restricted interests, and aloofness.) Even the concern about the MMR vaccine has probably driven parents to their doctors to rule out a diagnosis. Added to this enhanced awareness is the fact, Wing's fourth explanation, that children with autism have often been misdiagnosed as having, for example, extreme psychiatric conditions such as schizophrenia. Children with learning or other disabilities may also have had unrecognized autistic impairments. Fifth, the widening recognition of autism-like disorders has been matched, and probably also fuelled, by an explosion in services for these children – diagnostic, educational, family, occupational and residential.

The sixth possible cause of the increased diagnostic rates of autism relates to triggering factors, which includes the debate surrounding the MMR vaccine. The difficulty of completely disproving once and for all in the most confident of scientific terms that the vaccine is not a cause of autism is almost impossible. And so Wing, inevitably and perhaps frustratingly, has to conclude that 'it remains a possibility that MMR vaccination precipitates autism in a small number of children who are vulnerable'. Finally, Wing considers the evidence that there has indeed been a true increase in numbers of children with autism. She thinks probably not, and concludes that the best interpretation of the available evidence is that changes in diagnostic criteria and raised awareness explain 'most, if not all' of the higher incidence and prevalence of autism and its related disorders today.

The hunt for an explanation is important. But far more significant is what the increase in frequency means for those looking after children with autism. Fiona Scott's study of Cambridgeshire primary schools suggested that one out of every two schools includes at least one child with a diagnosis of autism. What provisions are in place for these children? The answer is too few.[24]

In a report published by the All Party Parliamentary Group on

Autism in 2001,[25] these service deficiencies were clearly defined – and they were considerable and far reaching. Autism costs the UK about £1 billion each year. The lifetime cost for each person with autism is almost £3 million. With better services for families, general practitioners, teachers and those working in widely varying parts of the social and health services, these high costs and the adverse quality of life they point to could be considerably ameliorated.

One positive consequence of the debate surrounding the safety of the MMR vaccine is that a spotlight has fallen on autism like never before. Books, news stories, and magazine articles about this condition have pushed themselves into the mainstream media, partly because the public's sensibility to autism has been heightened by the publicity surrounding the MMR vaccine. I am writing these words in Vancouver. I opened my newspaper (the *National Post*) this morning – Saturday, 15 May 2004 –only to see that the books section had a large headline: 'Autism from both sides of the glass wall.' Two more books had just been published about autism – *Through a Glass Wall: Journey into the Closed Off Worlds of the Autistic*, by Howard Buten, and *Songs of the Gorilla Nation: My Journey through Autism*, by Dawn Prince-Hughes. In the UK, Charlotte Moore's book, *George and Sam*, was published in 2004 to great acclaim. She described her experiences as a mother of three children, two of whom have autism. In *Not Even Wrong: Adventures in Autism*, Paul Collins reflects on his son's autistic illness. And Michael Fitzpatrick, a doctor and the father of a son with autism, has written a book called *MMR and Autism*. This new interest in autism is in every way to be welcomed. The challenge now is to persuade government to do something about it. The National Autistic Society is campaigning energetically to do so. In one especially telling advertisement published in newspapers in June 2004, the society's call for renewed attention ran like this: 'All thumbs, two left feet, blood out of a stone, ants in your pants, raining cats and dogs, eyes bigger than your belly, every cloud has a silver lining, eyes in the back of your head. How can someone with autism trust people when all they do is lie? People with autism take everything literally, so casual communication can be confusing and frightening.'

The imperative created by the now wide recognition of the increasing rate and impact of autism extends beyond immediate care. Research is important too. In the largest ever review of autism research conducted by the Medical Research Council (MRC) and published in December 2001, a comprehensive set of research strategies was developed to reorient autism studies. Given the complexity of the autism spectrum, a much more accurate and consistent definition of autism is required. Given the uncertainties about frequency and cause, a much better organized research network needs to be established. Given the now strong research interest across a range of psychological, psychiatric, basic scientific and behavioural disciplines, there needs to be a much more integrated approach to questions of cause and care than has existed up to now. And finally, given the plethora of ideas about what might trigger autism – toxins, infections, diet, genes, drugs and, yes, vaccines – more and better research is needed to confirm or refute what are often very weak signals of causal concern.[26]

A different, and in some ways a contrary, perspective on autism research was provided in 2004 by a group from the UK's Institute of Child Health, representing the National Autistic Society and Parents Autism Campaign for Education. Although academic researchers and those from the non-academic community agreed that priority areas for study were the possible environmental or genetic causes of autism and treatment interventions, there was one glaring omission from the responses of those they surveyed – a remarkably low priority was given to research on families and services, in terms of actual funding, ongoing research, and even apparent interest. The Institute of Child Health's report found that, surprisingly, no one had any overall picture of what research was being done in the field of autism. This absence of wider oversight makes sensible planning of research priorities impossible. The report recommended that such an oversight mechanism be established immediately.

What about research into the MMR vaccine? The MRC made general recommendations about research into causes, and it must have had MMR vaccination in mind when it called for independent replications of early and highly preliminary reports. But aside from concluding that current evidence did not support a link between the vaccine and autism, no particular studies were recommended. One can understand why. To set out the need for one or more pieces of research into the status of the MMR vaccine might have encouraged the idea that the MRC itself had doubts about the vaccine, which, of course, was not the case.

One of the few specialists who was brave enough to suggest specific work into the MMR vaccine was Lorna Wing. In 2002,[27] she wrote that

> Research on MMR vaccination is important . . . A study in which children were assessed regularly for any features of autistic spectrum disorder from birth until five years of age, when the diagnosis should be clear for most participants, would be of interest. It would not be ethical to demand that some were given MMR in one dose, some as separate injections and some not vaccinated at all, but the parents' own decisions are likely to vary. It would be appropriate to ensure the inclusion of some siblings of children with autistic spectrum disorders because they are known

to have a higher risk of developing such conditions . . . A cohort of this kind would provide the basis for a detailed study of a potential causal role for MMR vaccination and abnormalities of the immune system.

But how well placed is the UK, even with an additional £2.5 million provided by the Government, to deliver on the hopes of those concerned about a range of disorders affecting as many as one in 200 children? The answer, I believe, is that the UK is not well placed at all – indeed, we have an approach to autism research that is destined to fail. Consider, by contrast, the way autism research is organized in America.

In 2000, the US Congress passed the Children's Health Act, the most radical law imaginable to accelerate progress into understanding autism. The Act mandated the director of the foremost American research agency, the National Institutes of Health (NIH), to provide funds for creating no fewer than five centres of excellence in autism research. Each centre is to conduct laboratory and clinical research into the cause, diagnosis, early detection, prevention, control and treatment of autism. In doing this work, the Act makes it clear that centres must make available and accessible clinical services for patient care. In other words, here was an unprecedented political commitment to expand, intensify, and coordinate research into and services for children living with autism. The Act also established an Interagency Autism Coordinating Committee to oversee this remarkable effort.

US Government funding for autism research has increased dramatically. In 1997, $22 million was spent on studying autistic spectrum disorders. That figure had more than doubled to $52 million by 2000. In 2003, $70 million, an incredible figure by UK standards, was being devoted to autism research. These monies were spent on research, educational workshops, calls for innovative approaches to treatment, and ten collaborative programmes of excellence in autism. These collaborative programmes linked together dozens of investigators across twenty-six universities and involved over 2,000 families with children who had autism. These networks would allow urgent new public health questions to be answered quickly. The US Government planned to spend $60 million over five years to develop these programmes.

The centres of excellence in autism research, also mandated by the Children's Act of 2000, were part of the STAART programme – Studies to Advance Autism Research and Treatment. $12 million every year beginning in 2003 is to be invested in these operations. A critical element of this effort is to build in public participation at all levels, especially with the autism advocacy community. In 2003, the NIH announced that it planned to spend $65 million over five years for eight new centres across the US. Where is the equivalent programme of investment in the UK?

Britain has a great deal to learn from the American commitment to autism research, not only financially but also politically. Congress has recognized that autism is an increasing health issue for individuals and families. Politicians have been prepared to put their weight behind initiatives to strengthen services for and research into autism by increasing their year-on-year budgetary commitments. Not so in the UK, where government believes that a one-off lump sum of £2.5 million is sufficient to right the imbalances in knowledge and public understanding of this common and poorly understood disorder.

In March and April 2004, I wrote to John Reid, the UK Government's Secretary of State for Health, asking whether one positive benefit of the debate surrounding the alleged MMR vaccine–autism link might be a renewed commitment to autism research. I tried to draw attention to the American programme of escalating investment and its funding for specialist centres of research. I asked whether 'now might be a propitious moment to commit further funds to autism investigation'.

I received a reply from Lord Norman Warner, a Parliamentary Under Secretary of State.[28] He agreed that 'The Government recognizes the importance of encouraging further research into autistic spectrum disorders.' But he wrote that,

> Progress on developing research proposals is, of course, dependent on researchers being ready and able to take forward projects of major significance. Before considering whether we should issue any further ring-fenced funding for autism research, we would wish to have a clearer idea of what is being achieved by the funds provided to date, and whether other good quality research proposals can be funded as part of the MRC's mainstream research programme.

Sadly, the Government prefers to wait for scientists to knock randomly at its – or the MRC's – door rather than leading an effort to scale up autism research networks, as its American counterpart has done so successfully. To call this a missed opportunity would be an understatement. Resistance to long-term investment in autism research, among those charged with responsibility for the public's health, has encouraged families to create their own means to study the condition affecting their children. A good example of this kind of grassroots initiative is the Autism Intervention Research Trust, launched in 2003. This charity, which is closely associated with the UK's National Autistic Society, aims to fund reliable research into novel treatments for autism. Once again the history of autism – establishment neglect, followed by parental activism – is repeated.

CHAPTER 5

Can Measles Be Eradicated?

'It is a well-worn axiom, but not a perfect one, that the world is content with appearances. One should add, to make the axiom complete, that the world is never contented with, and often does not care about, and often is intolerant of, the substance.'

Measles is a hidden global catastrophe and a moral atrocity. These twin claims may seem like exaggerations. Sadly, they are not. About 3 million cases of measles are reported worldwide each year. But the correct figure – the 'substance' as opposed to the 'appearance' – is more like 30 million.[1] Roughly 98 per cent of the annual 600,000 or so deaths from measles take place in the poorest parts of the world, especially in sub-Saharan Africa and India. Yet well over 90 per cent of the money spent on the provision of measles vaccine is devoted to the richest countries of the world.[2] Measles is the most common vaccine-preventable disease of childhood. It is a major cause of preventable blindness. And, because of its associated complications, measles infection is probably responsible for more deaths among children than any other virus or bacterium. Global catastrophe? Moral atrocity? There are few more stark and tragic examples of human neglect.

In Africa, measles can sometimes seem like a completely different disease to the one we are used to seeing in the industrialized world. The virus can cause devastating outbreaks of infection with many more complications and far higher death rates than one would ordinarily expect. The reasons for the dramatically greater human impact of measles are not entirely clear. The large burden of urban migration and displaced peoples following wars and natural disasters, together with the effects of an underlying and expanding HIV epidemic, have all served to intensify the prevalence of the infection. HIV doubles or triples the risk of death in children with measles. Malnutrition lessens the chances that a child who contracts measles will recover. And the greater exposure that accompanies overcrowding, especially in large extended families living in the same space, escalates the spread of the virus and consequently the severity of the disease.

The absence of health-care services only adds to the difficulties. There is frequently no capacity within a less-developed country's rickety health system to respond to measles outbreaks, let alone the swathes of sick individuals the virus leaves behind. Efforts to introduce vaccination programmes may be thwarted by the poor quality of the 'cold chain' – a system of protections and procedures that is needed to maintain the low temperatures required for vaccine viability. It may even be true that some governments do not even perceive measles to be a serious problem. The international focus is presently on more fashionable diseases, such as HIV–AIDS, malaria, and tuberculosis, leaving little time for politicians and public health officials to focus attention and resources on measles.

In developing countries, the diagnosis of measles has to be made quickly and decisively to improve the chances of saving the child's life. A very simple clinical picture is used to identify an episode of this potentially fatal infection. A child is said to have measles if it has fever, a rash all over the body, plus *either* a cough *or* a runny nose *or* red eyes. This simple clinical approach means that few children with measles should be missed.

The course of the illness associated with measles virus infection can be extraordinarily severe. The rash can knit together to create a raised mat of red skin, which blackens and bleeds in the worst of cases. The lungs and throat become inflamed, producing a nasty cough and acute difficulty in breathing. The gut is affected too, causing massive diarrhoea, a crippling loss of essential protein, and preventing the absorption of remedial food and water. Weight loss is usual and only adds to the chances of death. The misery that follows infection often produces a refusal to eat and may turn the child away from breastfeeding – a vital lifeline to survival. Inflammation of the brain – encephalitis – although relatively infrequent, is another desperate sign of impending disaster.

The low physical state to which the child is reduced by measles only paves the way for further infections. Pneumonia kills more children with measles than any other single cause. Infections of the bowel will produce further diarrhoea and loss of protein. The mouth, palate, gums and lips may ulcerate, creating immense pain and distress. The eye, too, will develop ulcers, sometimes leading to blindness. The whole awful effect of measles is therefore to induce a state of agony for the child and parent alike.

Worse still, there is no specific treatment. The best that can be offered is a series of physical props, provided in the hope that the body will mount its own efforts to get rid of the virus. Food and fluid are mainstays. They are not easy to give. The consequences of the infection – mouth ulcers, extensive bowel disease, diarrhoea – all sap the last remaining sparks of motivation in the child to survive. If some food and water do go down, oxygen, antibiotics and a good dose of vitamin A may also help. Oxygen counters the effects of any developing pneumonia. Antibiotics are important because combined infections with other bacterial diseases can greatly add to the risk of death, sometimes doubling the chances of demise. Two oral doses of vitamin A have been shown to halve mortality rates and greatly diminish complications when given early in the course of infection. The result is that with good supportive care, death rates from measles can be reduced to between three and six children per 100 infected. This number remains a scar on vulnerable communities since, although the absolute frequency of infection is low, the total population of children affected is high because of the virus's rampant infectivity.

But measles can be controlled. The creation of a vaccine, as I described in Chapter 1, has transformed the impact of measles on human populations – or at least, on those populations that can afford the vaccine and that enjoy the commitment of their politicians to ensuring its widespread provision. Neither of these two conditions is true in many parts of the world today.

Less than complete immunization among a population can still seriously interfere with the measles virus's ability to spread. For example, vaccine coverage of 80 per cent or more can lengthen the gap between outbreaks of measles to four years or so. Fewer children will die if they do contract measles at these relatively low levels of coverage, perhaps because the intensity of their exposure to the virus is greatly diminished. Nevertheless, a real and permanent ending to measles virus circulation will require vaccine coverage in the order of 95 per cent. A truly formidable challenge.

It can be done. In 1997, the distinguished measles expert Heikki Peltola announced that measles had been eliminated from Finland.[3] He was not complacent about this achievement, recognizing that 'The threat of measles is not behind us, and we expect to see at least some cases in the years ahead,' most likely among those who had not been vaccinated or in those in whom the vaccine had failed.

There are huge economic incentives for those with the political power to eradicate measles from the world. According to one estimate, global measles eradication would save America between $500 million and $4 billion (at 1997 dollar rates). Taking the UK together with Canada, Denmark, Finland, the Netherlands, Spain and Sweden, over $600 million could possibly be saved by eradicating measles.[4] An added incentive for those contemplating a policy of global eradication is revealed by the debate launched after Wakefield's *Lancet* paper was first published. As the incidence of measles falls, so the public's perceptions of the benefits of vaccination also fall. And, rather more dangerously, so the damaging impact of advertising rare, even unproven, vaccination adverse events takes its toll on the public's confidence in vaccination policy. Eradication would therefore have the social value of eliminating not only measles, but also any small real, theoretical or imagined risk of vaccination and its adverse public impact.

Europe has a well-worked-out strategy for controlling measles. The continent may indeed come close to hitting its target of interrupting measles transmission by 2010. The difficulty that Europe faces is its fragmented nature. There are three Europes, not one. The first is what most people in the west think of as Europe – twenty-three nations that include the UK, Germany, France, Italy, Spain and so on. In this western Europe, the number of reported measles cases has declined from 229,447 in 1991 to 16,575 in 2001 – an impressive 93 per cent fall.

The second Europe is that made up by the newly independent states of the former Soviet Union (twelve countries, including the Russian Federation, Ukraine, Uzbekistan, Kazakhstan and Belarus). In these nations, the health-care infrastructure and resources to pay for vaccination are profoundly strained. Yet reported measles cases have fallen by 53 per cent, from 43,122 in 1991 to 20,402 in

2001 – a significant achievement by any standards. Most disappointing of all, however, has been the third Europe – those sixteen central and eastern states that include Turkey, Poland, Romania, the Czech Republic and Hungary. Here, reported measles cases were 31,585 in 1991, and remained at 30,782 in 2001 – a tiny 2.5 per cent decline. By 2005, irrespective of this great variation, all of the countries of Europe are expected to have devised national plans of action to control measles.

There are, therefore, considerable challenges ahead. The average annual reported measles incidence rate per 100,000 population over the most recently available five-year period[5] in the UK is a mere 0.2 cases. In western Europe, the worst measles offender is France (an alarming sixty-seven cases per 100,000 population), followed by Belgium (thirty-three cases), Switzerland (twenty-nine cases), San Marino (eighteen cases), and Italy (eighteen cases). In the newly independent states, the least effective measles control takes place in Tajikistan (twenty-three cases per 100,000 population), followed by Krygyzstan (sixteen cases), Azerbaijan (fourteen cases), Ukraine (thirteen cases), and Moldova (eleven cases). In central and eastern Europe, the measles scoreboard is led by Albania and Bosnia-Herzegovina (both thirty-seven cases per 100,000 population each), followed by Turkey (thirty-four cases).

These numbers put the furore over Wakefield's claims into its proper perspective. While fear surely did grip a part of the British population over the safety of the MMR vaccine, the actual impact of the debate has been marginal in its effects on measles incidence when set against the European backdrop. Indeed, the predicament of measles across the three Europes remains serious, substantial, and unresolved.

*

Measles has been in the sights of international health bureaucrats for at least a generation. In 1989, the World Health Assembly of the World Health Organization established the goal of reducing measles deaths by 90 per cent by 1995 compared with pre-immunization levels. The World Summit for Children adopted the target in 1990 of immunizing some 90 per cent of children against measles by 2000. Neither objective was met.

Against this background of failure, a landmark meeting was held in July 1996 between representatives of WHO, the Pan American Health Organization, and the US Centers for Disease Control and Prevention. The assembled experts wanted to decide once and for all whether measles could truly be eradicated from the world and, if so, what it would take to do so.

The mood among most of the participants was optimistic. Measles had largely been eliminated from the Americas and the UK. Eradication could be contemplated if the political and public health commitment was shown to be there. Measles eradication was certainly technically feasible and could build on what was then seen as the success of the effort to eradicate polio. The live vaccine used against measles should be sufficient to do the job. All that needed to be done was to increase the recommended vaccination schedule from a single jab to one providing all children with a second opportunity for measles immunization. This second opportunity was added to make sure that children who escaped measles vaccination through routine immunization services and those who were vaccinated but who failed to respond to the vaccine were protected against infection. A possible model immunization strategy for measles eradication was proposed. This three-tiered immunization policy had been very successful in the Americas for interrupting measles virus circulation: the so-called 'catch-up, keep-up, and follow-up' strategy.

The problem facing the would-be measles eradicators was, however, more difficult than any straightforward operational barrier. They wrote that:[6]

> The major obstacles to measles eradication are not technical but perceptual, political, and financial. Measles is often mistakenly perceived as a mild illness. This misperception, which is particularly prevalent in industrialized countries, can inhibit the development of public and political support for the allocation of resources required for an effective elimination effort. The disease burden imposed by measles should be documented, particularly in industrialized countries, so that this information can be used to educate parents, medical practitioners, public health workers and political leaders about the benefits of measles eradication.

The answer, then, lay in good public relations. The decision to eradicate came after a great deal of vacillation. Many critics of eradication policies had argued that measles was too contagious to be erased from the world. Or that the lack of an effective vaccine for children under nine months of age – when the mother's protective antibodies to measles also prevent the child's immune system from responding to the live virus vaccine – would always keep open a window of opportunity for measles to regain a foothold in human populations. (In developing countries, many children die from measles before they are twelve months old and so the earlier the vaccine can be given – at six to nine months, ideally – the better.) But the sheer scale of vaccination success was hard to ignore. In 1980, 2.5 million children died from measles infection. That figure had fallen to 924,000 deaths by 1995. Compared with the pre-vaccine era, when there were an estimated 6 million annual measles deaths, measles mortality had been slashed by about 85 per cent. A target date for eradication was provisionally set for somewhere between 2005 and 2010.

This enthusiasm continued. In May 2000, measles strategists convened at WHO's headquarters in Geneva to review their gradually developing plans to eliminate the virus. The epidemiology of measles seemed to be in WHO's favour. The virus was not evenly distributed throughout the world. Over 90 per cent of all measles deaths in 2000 took place in forty-five countries across Africa and Asia. And in 1999, only fourteen countries had measles vaccine coverage below 50 per cent: Afghanistan, Angola, Central African Republic, Chad, Congo, Democratic People's Republic of Korea, Democratic Republic of Congo, Djibouti, Equatorial Guinea, Ethiopia, Niger, Nigeria, Somalia and Togo. Success therefore depended on quickly ramping up immunization schedules from one dose of the vaccine to providing all children with a second opportunity for measles immunization. (Most developing countries outside the Americas use a single measles vaccine for routine immunization, not the MMR vaccine.) The first dose should be given at nine months of age through routine health services. Countries should then provide a second opportunity for children to be immunized later on. Vaccine coverage had to be greater than 90 per cent if elimination was to be achieved. But there was one unavoidable problem. Measles could never be WHO's top priority while polio remained a threat.

Perhaps because of this *realpolitik*, a discernible change of heart became apparent when a new joint plan was announced between WHO and the United Nations Children's Fund (UNICEF) in 2001.[7] The goal of the global measles strategic plan shifted to reduce the number of measles deaths by half by 2005. To be fair, eradication was not completely pushed off the agenda. WHO and UNICEF promised to convene a 'global consultation' in 2005 to 'assess the feasibility of global measles eradication'. (The current thinking at WHO is that this meeting may still take place at the end of 2005, although 2006 is also a possibility, since by then we will know whether the 2005 target has been reached.) Of course, feasibility had been considered once before, back in 1996. Why now a second time? The issues that had to be argued over were only partly technical:

> Several questions have to be answered before a decision is made on a new target for measles control. Some of them relate to the level of societal and political support for different goals . . . clearly, more information and experience are required before the decision on a measles eradication goal can be thoroughly assessed.

As 2005 drew nearer, pressure continued to be applied to WHO to scale up its efforts on measles. The World Health Assembly is WHO's parliament of 192 member governments. It meets annually in May. In 2003, it passed a resolution (WHA56.20) urging member states to implement fully the joint WHO–UNICEF strategic plan for measles mortality reduction. The Assembly also instructed WHO's new Director-General, Lee Jong-wook, to work with countries to strengthen national immunization services and to secure the necessary financial resources to implement the agency's ambitious measles strategy. These resources are estimated to be about $140 million annually between 2004 and 2008, one third of which must go towards paying for the vaccine itself.

Global progress was reviewed later that year in October. Over 200 experts gathered in Cape Town to plan ways to meet the 2005 goal of halving measles mortality compared with 1999 levels. They included Carol Bellamy, the executive director of UNICEF, signifying her organization's critical role in procuring and distributing vaccine supplies. 'The single leading reason for the continuing high global burden of measles', the meeting concluded, was the 'under-utilization of currently available safe, effective, and relatively inexpensive measles vaccine'.

Still, the prospects looked encouraging. A global network of over 600 laboratories across 150 countries was in place to ensure the rapid diagnosis of suspected measles cases. The number of these laboratories had doubled between 2002 and 2003. In the field, a policy of Reaching Every District (RED) had been put in place as the crucial foundation for saving children's lives. Immunization has to reach every village, measles surveillance has to be strengthened, and information about who has been vaccinated and when must be carefully collected. All in all, WHO and UNICEF believed that they were on track to meet their goal of halving measles deaths by the end of 2005 – the first global measles target that will ever have been successfully achieved.

An optimistic snapshot of progress was provided in January 2004. As the table below shows, there has been a decline in measles mortality by almost a third between 1999 and 2002:[8]

Region	1999 Estimated Deaths	2002 Estimated Deaths	Change (% decrease)
Africa	482,000	312,000	–170,000 (–35%)
South-East Asia	243,000	196,000	–47, 000 (–19%)
Eastern Mediterranean	104,000	71,000	–33,000 (–32%)
Others	40,000	35,000	–5,000 (–13%)
GLOBAL	869,000	614,000	–255,000 (–29%)

As these figures show, Africa is central to any serious effort to combat measles. Indeed, measles is the number one priority vaccine-preventable disease for the continent. The problem of measles in Africa can be solved. The major reduction of measles deaths from southern Africa in 2000 – across seven nations (South Africa, Botswana, Namibia, Zimbabwe, Swaziland, Malawi and Lesotho) – was an enormous achievement,[9] second only to clearing measles from the Americas. An incredible 24 million children aged between nine months and fourteen years of age were vaccinated from 1996 to 2000. That number represented over 90 per cent of all such children in these countries. This unparalleled mass effort cut measles cases from 60,000 to just 117 in four years. Most encouragingly of all, these advances were achieved in regions of very high HIV–AIDS prevalence, especially in Botswana, South Africa, and Zimbabwe. Measles is more severe in children with HIV–AIDS and the risks of contracting a fatal secondary infection are far worse. Also importantly, there were no significant adverse effects from vaccination.

To be sure, there are tough challenges ahead. In September 2003, in the Jamalpur district of Bangladesh, three children who had been immunized died. The reason was a contaminated supply of the vaccine – a 'programmatic error' that demanded quick investigation and strong reassurance through the local media in order to maintain confidence in the immunization campaign. Such unplanned tragedies are bound to recur. New strains of measles virus are occasionally reported, thanks to better surveillance, complicating diagnostic and prevention efforts.[10] Unusual clinical presentations of measles infection, or infections that do not produce typical symptoms, may mislead even vigilant health workers, enabling measles virus to escape detection and elimination.[11] As the incidence of measles falls around the world, an increasingly important source of the virus that could reinfect very young non-immune children (infants less than nine months old) will be hospitals. Preventing these 'nosocomial' outbreaks of measles will present a difficult problem as we come close to eradicating the virus,[12] as will the expanding number of displaced peoples whose inevitably absent health services will make it almost impossible to reach the kind of vaccine coverage necessary to stop further measles outbreaks.[13]

But the immediate short-term obstacle remains polio. At the Cape Town meeting in 2003, experts warned that unless polio eradication was completed successfully, it would be difficult to achieve global measles goals. And yet polio is proving harder to eradicate than first thought. Nigeria suspended vaccinations during 2004 in some regions, following fears that the vaccine was being used to control the fertility of its Islamic populations. New outbreaks of polio have been seen there and in twenty other African nations, mainly through importation. Five times as many children in central and west Africa were paralysed in 2004 compared with 2003. 'There is no question that the [polio] virus is spreading at an alarming pace', said Dr David Heymann, WHO's special representative for polio eradication. India also continues to struggle in its final push towards eradication.[14]

After all the technical issues have been resolved, and after all the lobbying to secure political commitment has been undertaken, victory over measles depends on the trust of the public. And this is why scares such as that sparked by Wakefield's claims are so damaging. Writing recently from UNICEF's headquarters in New York, Heidi Larson, seemingly with Wakefield at the forefront of her mind, warned that:

> To achieve, maintain, and sustain successful immunization pro-
> grammes it is necessary to win and keep the trust of the public.
> This is more difficult to do than previously, because there are

more sources of information, they are more decentralized (the internet), and less scrutinized. The result is that small groups with high motivation and commitment can deliver their message easier, even if the message has no merit. Marginalized anti-immunization groups have taken advantage of this.

The critical question still remains at the beginning of the twenty-first century: can measles be eradicated from the world?[15] The answer is yes. This is the course that should be set when experts gather in 2005 or 2006. Measles can be eradicated from the world by 2015 – only a decade away. There will be tremendous difficulties. Leave aside the fact that the problems facing polio eradication are bound to spill over into delays in measles elimination. There are three important and substantial short-term blocks facing those who want to rid the world of measles. All three of these obstacles are currently under-estimated by the many public health enthusiasts for measles eradication. They are not impossible to overcome, but they require far more sophisticated thought than they have received to date.

The first and by far the most important barrier is simply political. It makes sense to argue for a once-and-for-all eradication policy because the political commitment that this approach will demand is time limited. If a less ambitious goal is set – for example, a more rigorously defined mortality reduction target beyond 2005 – success will depend on inevitably shifting long-term political commitments. Still, the reality is that the seriousness with which governments take measles today varies so greatly that any short to medium-term plan for aligning all nations in the same direction concerning measles eradication is going to be tough to deliver. One only has to look at some of the world's richest countries that have surprisingly low rates of vaccine coverage – Germany, 75 per cent; Japan, 68 per cent;

Austria, 60 per cent; and Italy, 50 per cent, all of which, not surprisingly, continue to experience frequent measles outbreaks. Given competing global public health priorities (HIV–AIDS, malaria and tuberculosis, in particular), it seems that there is little appetite (or money) for yet another disease eradication initiative.

One initiative could do much to win support for worldwide measles eradication – the Global Alliance for Vaccines and Immunization (GAVI), which was launched in 2000. GAVI aims to advocate for the wider use of vaccines and to expand the capacity of national immunization services. It is a consortium representing WHO, UNICEF, the World Bank, the Bill and Melinda Gates Foundation, the Vaccine Fund and many other partners. One of its most important roles is to build consensus around global immunization efforts, of which measles must be its single most important priority.

And yet, astonishingly, GAVI has, until recently, been failing children at risk of measles. GAVI describes its mission as one that is 'focused on increasing access to vaccines among children in poor countries'. But it has not lived up to this fine statement of principle. In 2003, GAVI announced that it endorsed the WHO/UNICEF measles immunization strategy. Carol Bellamy, then chair of GAVI's board and also Executive Director of UNICEF, said that, 'we have the opportunity to save well over 2 million young lives using a proven strategy. Measles immunizations have saved the lives of over 130,000 children in Africa this year. We must now build on this success and ensure that every child is adequately vaccinated and protected against measles.'

Later that year, UNICEF urged GAVI to invest $50 million ($10 million per year over five years) to prevent children from dying needlessly from measles. Despite GAVI's earlier rhetoric, when it came to providing hard cash its board members demurred. Some did not want to pay for an old, tried-and-tested vaccine. They were more interested in the modish enterprise of developing new technologies and vaccines – not for measles, but for diseases such as hepatitis B. In response, measles control advocates drew up a 'measles investment case' that was discussed by GAVI in May 2004. The benefits of the proposed funding were made explicitly clear: $50 million would save 1.84 million children from dying unnecessarily across 35 African countries. Again, the board declined to act, instead requesting pedantic clarifications that were easily answerable there and then. Only in July 2004, did GAVI accede to this request for investment. The feeling among those closest to efforts to eradicate measles is that the World Bank and the Gates Foundation did not want GAVI to invest in measles. These organizations seem opposed to mass vaccination campaigns and are unlikely to support calls for global measles eradication. This reticence is shameful given the many thousands of lives that can be saved.

A second barrier concerns the present live-attenuated vaccine. Coverage rates of over 90 per cent are needed to achieve effective measles control. Needle-based immunization programmes present many difficulties. Most importantly, they introduce new risks of blood-borne infections, such as hepatitis B and HIV, being transmitted through the use of the needles themselves. Although the introduction of autodisposable syringes (needles and syringes that can only be used once) has greatly reduced the risk of disease transmission, their exclusive use in the vaccination programmes of developing countries has uncovered another major challenge – assuring the appropriate disposal of used immunization equipment. The use of autodisposable syringes in routine immunization services and mass campaigns has caused an acute worsening of a longstanding problem: what to do about hazardous toxic waste.

The delivery of measles vaccine through aerosols may be one means of avoiding the risk of transmitting blood-borne infections.[16] The vaccine can be delivered through a face mask by means of a spray generated by passing pressurized air from an electrically powered compressor through a solution of the vaccine. These tiny particles of vaccine land in the lungs, providing a painless, quick, non-invasive and practical means for non-health-care personnel to run a vaccination campaign successfully and cheaply. WHO envisages that an aerosolized version of the measles vaccine will not be licensed until 2007, reaching the field only by 2009.

A more contentious area concerns the nature of the vaccine itself. Is the vaccine currently used both alone and as a component of MMR good enough for the job of eradicating measles? Many experts believe that it is. But the vaccine's effectiveness is only 90–95 per cent. It is ineffective in children under nine months of age. Almost all measles experts agree that if a way could be found to protect these young infants, who are at the greatest risk of harm from the virus, eradication efforts would be greatly assisted. Indeed, some would say that measles will be impossible to control in the crowded cities of Africa and India unless such a vaccine becomes available. One example illustrates this challenge only too well.[17] In an orphanage in India in 1996, six children fell ill with measles. One was eleven months old, one seven months old, and four were four months of age or less. None of these infants had been vaccinated against measles. No child died, although one did develop encephalitis.

The perfect measles vaccine would be given in very early infancy – between three and six months of age – and it should induce long-lasting immunity in over 95 per cent of vaccinees. The existing live vaccine does not meet these requirements. In literature discussing this vaccine, words such as 'drawbacks' and 'minor flaws' are commonly used. Scientists write about the need for 'an improved vaccine for global measles control'.[18] One of the difficulties caused by the Wakefield affair is the understandable reluctance among public health officials to admit these imperfections. The goal has been to restore confidence in the MMR vaccine, not to point out its shortcomings.

Yet, from a global perspective, problems there are. The live vaccine is unstable at ambient temperatures. A vaccine that could survive the extreme weather conditions of the tropics would be a huge step forward. A vaccine that was able to evade the neutralizing activity of the mother's natural antibodies, which are transferred to the fetus towards the end of pregnancy, would be an additional advantage. There is continuing concern that infection with HIV induces a state of profound immunosuppression that might render a live vaccine dangerous, although to date there is little evidence to suggest that this risk is significant. The existing vaccine seems to produce lower levels of protection than infection with naturally occurring measles virus. And finally, if the world did ever come very close to complete measles eradication, the use of a live vaccine could maintain and not extinguish the circulation of measles in the community, leaving open the remote possibility that a vaccine strain which had lost some of its attenuation could escape and pose a serious danger to health.

There are other benefits that would come from a better vaccine. Today's measles vaccine was produced in what would now be considered a very rough and ready way – by the serial passage of the virus through one cell culture after another (see Chapter 1). While this process has been extremely successful in securing a safe and effective vaccine, this kind of attenuation is uncontrolled. As a result, we know very little about the molecular basis underlying human immunity to measles. What scientists would like to be able to do is to build a non-replicating (a 'dead') measles vaccine, one for which we understand precisely the genetic and immunological basis for the protection afforded by the vaccine. As the virologists Gregory Atkins and Louise Cosby have written,

> We believe that there is a case for the development of a new and safer recombinant vaccine to replace the current MMR vaccine, which is not capable of extensive replication in the host [human being], and which can be manipulated to induce protective immunity in a controlled manner.

For these reasons, many new and very different measles vaccines are being investigated in animals. Some are even coming close to being studied in human trials. This important work should be urgently expanded if we are to have any serious chance of eradicating measles. The effort to discover a new vaccine does not mean that MMR is unacceptably flawed. It is a testament to the success of the MMR vaccine that we are within reach of extinguishing measles from the world within a decade. Yet a new vaccine that can overcome the weaknesses of the present live attenuated virus vaccine would greatly facilitate progress towards measles eradication.

There are significant hurdles that any new measles vaccine will have to clear before it can be widely introduced. It will have to be proven in clinical trials to be better than the existing live vaccine. It is bound to be costly. And the upheaval in altering global immunization strategies will be vast. One further strange twist to this story is that we may not want to end vaccination completely.[19] Measles immunization seems to confer benefits that have nothing to do with eliminating the measles virus itself. Measles vaccination appears able to enhance resistance to other infections, perhaps by broadly stimulating the immune system. A further small, but tangible, risk is that eradicating measles would leave the world vulnerable to bioterrorist attack – a not so fanciful threat in today's age.[20]

There is one final question that advocates for measles eradication must consider.[21] This concerns the value of a 'vertical' programme of action directed at one disease. It could be argued that a successful eradication programme will encourage more donor aid and foreign direct investment into poorer nations. Success begets success. But a far more compelling possibility is that there are dangers of singling out one disease from all others.

Perhaps a broader perspective is needed in which to view the quest to obliterate measles. About 10 million children die each year.[22] Six countries – India, Nigeria, China, Pakistan, the Democratic Republic of Congo and Ethiopia – account for half of all deaths seen in children under five years of age. Under-nutrition is a critical underlying factor behind many of these deaths. Over half are attributable to malnutrition. Children commonly have multiple concurrent illnesses, not one easily definable condition, such as measles. Pneumonia and diarrhoea are frequently still associated with childhood mortality. Drinking contaminated water, together with poor conditions of hygiene and sanitation, contributes to 1.5 million child deaths each year. If breastfeeding does not take place in early infancy, the chances of dying can rise seven-fold.

Indeed, almost two-thirds of total childhood deaths in the world could be prevented with known interventions. These interventions – for example, good maternal care – are simply not available. The effort to control, eliminate, and finally to eradicate measles is a vitally important global goal. It provides the lever with which to implement an even higher priority – to attack child mortality by looking at the lives of children in their widest context. This means thinking about something quite mundane. How do we strengthen every country's health system – expanding the number of trained health-care workers, improving the supply of all essential drugs and vaccines, increasing the capacity to obtain the best and most accurate information about local needs, and creating basic health services in villages, districts and regional centres? As Jennifer Bryce, a child health specialist with decades of experience in some of the poorest regions of the world, wrote in 2003, 'child survival interventions are not reaching the children who need them most'. It is hard to understand why and it is unacceptable to allow this situation to continue. Measles eradication provides our best hope to make a difference for the most vulnerable group of human beings in the world today.

CHAPTER 6

The Manufacture of Fear

'In abstruse matters the minority always sees better than the majority, while the majority sees better in things that are evident.'

I began this book by suggesting that there is a malaise in the way that we, as a society, discuss scientific controversies. The debate (or, better still, débâcle) over the MMR vaccine is one very good, if extreme, example of this malaise. Such a proposition is not especially controversial, except, perhaps, among journalists, who I think would vigorously defend the work they do in reporting these kind of disputes. And yet those who study and write about the media seem to readily acknowledge that journalism is itself suffering a malaise. Are these two phenomena related? I believe that they are.

Vincent Campbell, in his book *Information Age Journalism*,[1] argues that in the twenty-first century 'the status and nature of journalism, perhaps surprisingly, is unclear . . . The more one looks around at journalism across the globe, the more one sees the notion of crisis, or at the very least, notions of uncomfortable transition, apparent in many nations.' The reasons he gives for this uncertainty are diverse. Audiences for news are declining. Media ownership is coalescing around a few dominant global corporations, diminishing pluralism and perhaps even eroding the possibility for muscular political debate. The dramatic expansion of digital television and the internet has been the driving force behind a flourishing entertainment industry, while at the same time fragmenting and reducing the importance of news. This shift away from forums for serious public discussion has led some news media to exaggerate or emphasize the sensationalist elements of a story, in the hope of successfully introducing entertainment into old-fashioned news reporting. The crisis within journalism is therefore one of identity. The notion of journalism's purpose as being socially valuable, creating a space for public deliberation as an arm of democracy, has been gradually giving way, so the pessimists would argue, to the idea of journalism as purely a business among many others in an age of aggressively competing information sources and media outlets.

In Britain, this view has been strengthened substantially by John Lloyd, in his book *What the Media are Doing to Our Politics*. Lloyd is a distinguished reporter and editor. He takes the crisis over British journalism during the Iraq war in 2003 as his starting point for a raucous critique of his colleagues. Lloyd argues that the media has become 'destructive . . . of public communication and of democratic practise'. Nothing less than 'a renewal of the values and tasks' of journalism will do. He suggests that his fellow editors rarely act as agents of social responsibility. They prefer comment to fact, scandal and revelation to detailed and subtle writing and conflict or satire to analytical and explanatory current affairs. In his view, the ideal of 'non-polemical Enlightenment' has been abandoned. I think Lloyd goes too far. The media should pose hard, sometimes abrasive, questions. They should expose failure. A clash of opinions, well managed, is a valid way to search for truth. But he is correct when he writes that:

One reason why journalism is unpopular, especially with publicly accountable people like politicians, scientists, medical workers, and public officials, is that the reporters and the commentators keep popping up to slam them . . . many public figures thus conclude that journalists don't believe in anything but slamming people.

Science, public, news and media – a malaise, wrapped up in a crisis, all within a metamorphosis. The relationship between scientists and the public is at an all-time low. Science is no longer seen as a source of technological solutions to the everyday problems of life. It is a cause of pervasive social anxiety. Science is struggling through a thickening climate of suspicion, one that is now inscribed across our culture in a thousand different ways. Take just one recent and very powerful example – Margaret Atwood's *Oryx and Crake*, a novel describing an all too possible dystopia of technological bravado scarred by a series of unanticipated consequences, which was published to critical triumph in 2003 and subsequently short-listed for that year's Booker Prize and the 2004 Orange Prize for Fiction. It is an emblem of a science that contains within it a seed of evil.

Atwood begins *Oryx and Crake* with a quote by Jonathan Swift – 'my principal design was to inform you, and not to amuse you.' Her story opens after some kind of apocalypse. The narrator, Snowman, lives in a tree, over a beach of 'ground-up coral and broken bones'. He looks back and describes how he has arrived at this point. Atwood weaves Snowman's flashbacks into his present efforts to find food, since, only a few weeks after the 'Great Rearrangement', he is slowly starving to death. Atwood has created a time zone for her characters in which genetic technologies have enabled the invention of an animal called the pigoon. Snowman's father, who worked as a 'genographer', had been engaged in a project to grow an assortment of foolproof human-tissue organs in a transgenic knockout pig host – organs that would transplant smoothly and avoid rejection, but would also be able to fend off attacks by opportunistic microbes and viruses, of which there were more strains every year.

This is a novel replete with technical jargon, opening doors to catastrophic futures, and situating familiar technologies – such as vaccination – in a strange and sinister context. The pigoon could grow five or six kidneys at a time. It was programmed to mature rapidly and could be customized according to need. Snowman's father was a genius. He perfected wrinkle-free skin. He had discovered a way to grow human brain cortex in a pigoon – ostensibly to treat degenerative neurological diseases, an advance that comes back quite literally to stalk his son.

Crake is introduced as a brilliant biologist, trained at the Watson-Crick Institute (Harvard has, by this time, 'drowned'). He had created new forms of human being – the Crakers. Their skin oozes citrus to repel mosquitoes. Wounds are healed by the sonic vibrations of their cat-like purring. Children grow into adults quickly and their digestion has been re-engineered to make them herbivorous. Crake believes that he has deleted the cluster of neurons that creates God in our minds. His project is called Paradice. Crake's father had been murdered because he discovered a plan to create new diseases and spread them via vitamin pills. Now Crake is employed at a special compound called RejoovenEsense to create Crakers. He spends his time sculpting human embryos, enhancing immune systems, and inserting genetic programmes to bring about death at thirty. According to Crake, this is a type of immortality, a life lived in the absence of fear. The Crakers were designed to exist in communities with no claims on territory, no hierarchies, no marriage, no divorce – and no jokes.

Apocalypse comes from one of Crake's other inventions, sold around the world by Oryx. The BlyssPluss Pill will end war, stamp out contagious disease, and deal with over-population. The pill will eliminate all hazards and the Crakers will repopulate the earth to create a superior world. Crake intends to take up where the covert project his father once started left off. He orchestrates a massive global airborne infectious epidemic (a super-measles?) that causes riots, looting and fires – and cataclysmic waves of human death.

Snowman not unreasonably believes that 'some line has been crossed, some boundary transgressed'. He asks, 'How much is too much, how far is too far?' But his father had seen these events as inevitable: 'This is where it ends up . . . once things get going,' he says at one point. Atwood's theme is summed up by Crake, who sees how fragile and contingent civilization truly is. All that is needed to destroy what we presently take for granted is a break in the line of history. Such a dislocation could be achieved by removing, at a single stroke, one generation. This is exactly what Crake tries to do, vaccinating his friend, Snowman, and creating new human forms – the Crakers – to do a better job than we had done before. Here, symbolically, is the great flood story retold, revised, and envisioned some time in the mid twenty-first century. Paradice the Ark, and Snowman Noah – Crake is indeed acting like an omnipotent power when he asks Snowman, 'Would you kill someone you loved to spare them pain?' Sometimes the only answer, horrifying as it is, Atwood seems to be saying, is yes.

The literature of dystopia is not new. From Samuel Butler's anti-technological *Erewhon* (1872) to Ray Bradbury's meditation on censorship in *Fahrenheit 451* (1953), portrayals of future societies in which something has gone badly wrong have become common vehicles to sum up our fears and hopes about the future. Dystopias are not only representations of imperfect societies. They also signify cultures in which evil has somehow become internalized into ordinary everyday life. The twenty-first century has brought with it something different: a new wave of anti-biological and disease-ridden dystopias. Margaret Atwood, for example, stressed that with *Oryx and Crake* she was writing speculative fiction – 'possible futures, not inevitable ones' – not science fiction: 'it invents nothing we haven't already invented or started to invent.'

Today, the pivot between scientists and the public is the scientific journal. The journal is the means by which all serious researchers must report their findings to their colleagues. It is also a source for journalists, who translate these technical documents into stories for a wider readership. Scientists cannot survive unless they publish. And the process and pecking order of publication is steeply hierarchical. There is nothing egalitarian about science. Journals carry reputations based upon their longevity, their impact, the fame of their editors (past and present), the speed of their publishing, and their visibility in whichever community the author wishes to be most revered by. Editors of scientific and medical journals mediate this process and are both loved and hated according to their willingness to give space to the hopeful investigator. Authors will try almost any trick to get published. I have been offered money and gifts, the promise of lavish hospitality, the guarantee of an award by a prestigious college, society and institution, and even riches for the publisher. Editors, who must try to avoid seductions both material and physical, rely on the imperfect process of peer-review to assist their decisions. But it is the editor who must take final responsibility for the fate of a research paper. Acceptance brings credibility and publicity to the author (and, ideally, to the editor and the journal). Rejection brings frustration, even anger (but, usually and thankfully, to the author only). The truth is that almost nothing will impede publication in one of the many thousands of journals that exist today but the want of a stamp (or perhaps a mouse). Good editors should have few friends, and those friends they do have should either be mad or dead.

When Thomas Wakley founded the *Lancet* in 1823, he wished to provide 'a work that would convey to the Public, and to distant Practitioners as well as to Students in Medicine and Surgery, reports of the Metropolitan Hospital Lectures'. Wakley duly published lectures by the great (and by today's standards rather dangerous) surgeons and physicians of his time. He published case reports gathered from England and the continent. The *Lancet* would be, under Wakley's direction, 'a complete Chronicle of current Literature'. Today we call this miscellany of clinical material 'research'. The word 'research' represents scientific shorthand for a vast range of different types of study, from the clinical trial of a new drug among 50,000 patients, to the humble clinical lesson learned from the 'case report' of a single patient. This diversity of approaches to a particular clinical problem is confusing. Not all evidence in the scientific literature is equally likely to be true. As the respected epidemiologists David Grimes and Ken Schulz have written, 'understanding what kind of study has been done is a prerequisite to thoughtful reading of research'.[2] This lesson in literacy is forgotten by some scientific editors and many journalists.

The Grimes and Schulz dictum is certainly appropriate when considering the status of Andrew Wakefield's 1998 *Lancet* paper. His was a study leaning much more towards the case report category of research than the clinical trial. By assembling twelve cases, Wakefield and his colleagues were attempting to draw preliminary conclusions about the existence of a new syndrome – the linkage of a peculiar type of bowel disease to autism. Oddly, some of the parents of these children and their doctors had noticed – nothing more – that the condition of the child seemed to deteriorate after they had received the MMR vaccine. This observation carried no statistical validity whatsoever. It was merely a signal that Wakefield took to fashion a hypothesis deserving of further study. This is frequently what happens in science. And it was indeed studied – and found to be wanting, at least according to research in large populations. But by then it was too late to dissuade people by repeating that the original *Lancet* report had raised only the weakest of signals of concern. We failed to convey the fragility of this signal to wider news media that were clamouring for answers, although, in mitigation, I would argue that we had not anticipated Wakefield fuelling this clamour by calling for the MMR vaccine to be split into its component parts – and the adverse public reaction was oddly confined to the UK.

Irrespective of the debate surrounding the original report – and the fact is that given what we know now about the circumstances surrounding the conduct of this work and its consequences for public health, it would have been better if it had not been published in the form that it was, with the MMR vaccine so prominently identified – the outcome was little less than an epidemic of fear. While the Government accused the media (including the *Lancet*) of stirring up an unnecessary panic, the media pointed to a wider crisis of trust in science and government advice. But the story of the MMR vaccine is not unique in the annals of medical misinformation.

'Has the health-effect of "passive smoking" been overestimated?' So ran the banner headline on the home page of British American Tobacco's website in May 2003. A click would have taken you to a summary of the company's views on the supposed dangers of environmental tobacco smoke. And then the surprise. The company concludes that: 'A very large new study of thousands of Californian adults, published in May 2003, in the *BMJ*, has found no increases in risk between environmental tobacco smoke exposure at home and the diseases of lung cancer, coronary heart disease and chronic obstructive pulmonary disease.' The study, it continued, 'confirms that many of the estimates of the risks of public smoking are overstated in the extreme . . . We believe the study illustrates that calls for bans on public smoking cannot be justified.'

The confident repudiations of a long-held scientific consensus that passive smoking kills stemmed from a paper published in the *British Medical Journal* by Dr James Enstrom and Dr Geoffrey Kabat.[3] Enstrom is a researcher at the school of public health at the University of California, Los Angeles; Kabat is an associate professor in the department of preventive medicine at the State University of New York – both respectable institutions. Their findings were extraordinary. They caused a storm of protest. And the *BMJ* was not spared the criticism of its enraged readers. After trawling data on 118,000 adults between 1959 and 1998, information that is held by the highly reputable American Cancer Society, the two doctors found no significant risks for men or women 'never smokers' who were married to 'ever smokers'. Any association between passive smoking and heart disease or lung cancer was 'considerably weaker than generally believed'.

In an unusually long conflict-of-interest statement, Enstrom and Kabat admitted receiving funds from the tobacco industry but claimed that 'they are both lifelong non-smokers whose primary interest is an accurate determination of the health effects of tobacco'. Had the *BMJ* been captured by the tobacco industry? Had its editors scored a massive own goal against the interests of public health? The British Medical Association, owners of the *BMJ*, clearly thought so. They called the *BMJ* study 'fundamentally flawed' and the data 'inadequate'. The American Cancer Society declared itself 'appalled'.

The media inadvertently buttressed the tobacco industry's position by portraying the controversy as a genuine scientific debate about the risks of passive smoking. The echoes of the MMR episode were uncanny. To the *BMJ*'s credit, their website provided an opportunity for an impassioned debate about not only the research but also the *BMJ*'s judgement in publishing work that clearly undermined every public health message doctors try to get across about smoking. The fallout was not pretty. Correspondents called for the paper to be retracted and for a public inquiry to be convened. The *BMJ*'s editors were pilloried for doing the dirty work of the tobacco industry. The *BMJ* was accused of becoming a comic among medical journals.

I would defend the *BMJ* and its editors. Medical journals are not instruments of public health policy. They are highly specialized newspapers. And if they are good at what they do, they will occasionally challenge received opinion, as all newspapers do. That is a good thing.[4] Given the intense media scrutiny of medical research, scientists are now under escalating pressure – from their funders, their institutions and journalists themselves – to think carefully and imaginatively about how their findings might be best communicated to the public. This concern for wider publicity has introduced a perverse and sometimes damaging set of incentives into medical research. If you are a charity that funds research, for example, your prosperity depends upon public donations. Such donations, in turn, depend upon the impression that the money being given will produce results of benefit to those living with the disease and whom the charity champions. The incentive for the charity to exaggerate the importance of new research is therefore great, since a high public profile is vital if it is to sustain its income. An example of this unfortunate confluence of interests is starkly apparent today in cancer research.[5] The outcome for the public is falsely raised expectations about cancer treatments and prevention.

Yet when controversies do arise, some scientists cry foul. Several years ago, the *Lancet* was embroiled in a dispute about the effectiveness of screening mammography to detect early cases of breast cancer. We had published a paper questioning the basis of the national breast cancer screening programme. The study was done by experienced scientists, but their findings incensed cancer specialists.[6] I took part in one radio debate with a leading British cancer researcher who was employed by a cancer charity that had no compunction in promoting preliminary research findings in the media as major breakthroughs or potential cures. He was indignant because I had given oxygen to a study that he clearly believed was flawed. He argued that my duty was to shore up public health messages about the importance of screening for breast cancer. He thought that I was irresponsible for publishing anything that challenged the value of screening. If this debate had to take place at all, he said, it should have been held in private, away from the public gaze and among scientists only.

Even if one believes in closing down debate rather than opening it up, which I do not, the idea that research can be discussed in secret is simply untenable today. Somehow, somewhere, and by someone, work of this kind will escape all efforts to control its disclosure. Surely it is better to lead the debate with passion and evidence than to chase after it in bitterness and exhortation. Many scientists may not agree. They fear that the media, and so the public, misinterpret research – for example, about animal experimentation, nanotechnology, or genetically modified foods – and trigger avalanches of anxiety from a few innocent snowflakes of concern. As Lord Robert May, the President of the Royal Society, has pointed out, the consequence of these confrontations is that the public gets 'caught in a confusing crossfire'.[7]

The occasionally adolescent relationship between scientists and journalists (and I include myself somewhere in the middle in this maladroit dance) was explored in the landmark House of Lords Select Committee on Science and Technology report entitled *Science and Society*, published in February 2000. The inquiry that preceded its publication captured much of the new thinking about science in the public realm, which had been slowly emerging during the previous few years. One of the reasons why this report was so important was simply this – that for the first time in recent memory all parties in the debate about how scientific issues are dealt with in the public sphere came together to agree that the status quo was no longer an option.

Their lordships concluded that 'Society's relationship with science is in a critical phase.' Public interest in science was high. Ninety per cent of the public expressed an avidity for new medical discoveries, for example, compared with only 66 per cent who were interested in sport. But public confidence in the advice provided by government scientists had been 'rocked' by the errors surrounding human risks from bovine spongiform encephalopathy. In one survey cited by the committee, and one that clearly had a powerful influence on its thinking, only 5 per cent of people had confidence in government scientists. Confidence was substantially higher (but still low, at 42 per cent) for scientists working in universities. These negative feelings about some groups of scientists seemed to be creating a lack of trust among the public concerning science more generally. Added to which was a social trend towards the questioning of all authority, not merely that bound up with science. If scientists were going to seek wider public support for what they did, they needed to work a great deal harder to understand and take account of why people felt like they did about science. Simply bludgeoning the public with facts, advice and reassurances would do nothing to restore trust.

This corrosion of trust, which is now endemic in society, has persuaded scientists to come out of their laboratories and talk to the public. In the select committee's more diplomatic language, there was now 'a new mood for dialogue'. In 2000, various levers were at the disposal of scientists to engage the public. The Committee on the Public Understanding of Science (COPUS) was formed in 1986 as a joint venture between the Royal Society, the Royal Institution and the British Association for the Advancement of Science. The Medical Research Council, the science museums and other funding bodies, such as the Wellcome Trust, all had important parts to play. Funding organizations could, for example, encourage the scientists they invested in to share their research findings with the public, rewarding those who did so. Scientists, in the select committee's view, had to shed their scepticism about colleagues who appeared, sometimes regularly, in the media. An austere disdain for media celebrity among scientists remains to this day. One only has to look at the way Susan Greenfield, who currently runs the Royal Institution, has been criticized for what some see as her courting of journalists at the expense, so it is alleged, of her work as a scientist.

Indeed, the public are no longer happy to be the passive recipients of scientific advice, whether over the safety of vaccinations or any other technology. The House of Lords committee described this different attitude as 'a new assertiveness on the part of the public'. The institutions of government and science needed radical change to go beyond the then preferred token event-based initiatives, such as citizen's juries and consensus conferences. There needed to be continuous and sustainable input into research organizations, learned institutions, and policy-making bodies from diverse groups in society. To put it more bluntly, 'In modern democratic conditions, science like any other player in the public arena ignores public attitudes and values at its peril.' Openness was the key idea behind change, and inclusivity in decision-making the way to bring change about.

The most difficult area for the select committee was how it should deal with the media. Many scientists and public health officials were – and still are – deeply unhappy about the way journalists handle science and medical news. They feel that their subject is trivialized, misreported, distorted, taken out of context or simply treated with utter disrespect. Given this widely prevalent hostility, the committee approached the matter carefully. It began with praise, noting that popular science journalism was 'flourishing' and 'thriving' in response to a strong public demand for science news. It divided science writing into two kinds – first, writing done by specialist science correspondents, and second, that done by news, politics or environment reporters who have little scientific background. The second group, the committee argued, rather acidly, was 'subject to a very different set of values and criteria'.[8]

There were several crucial points to understand about news reporting, which scientists either did not know or ignored, according to the select committee. Journalists are journalists, not public health advocates. It would be wrong to think that editors of newspapers or news programmes on radio and television are not concerned about accuracy. They are. But they are also concerned about delivering stories that are compelling in human terms – stories that make important subjects interesting. And they want those stories to be balanced. It is this notion of balance that causes scientists so much difficulty. News organizations commonly like to present at least two (opposing) sides to any issue. They are concerned not to be seen as biased in their news reports by giving only one side of the story. But for the scientist, giving equal weight to two opposing points of view may give too much time and credibility to a minority interest. The meaning of 'balance' for the journalist and scientist is very different, and has so far been irreconcilable.

Given these conflicting cultures of science and journalism, the

House of Lords Select Committee called for a 'sea change' in science. But not in journalism. About media coverage of science, the committee was more pragmatic:

> While it sometimes makes for public dialogue in terms which are unsatisfactory to some of the players, this is better than no dialogue at all. Scientists cannot expect special treatment from the media; they must take the rough with the smooth . . . Scientists must therefore learn to work with the media as they are.

Once again, the key was open and positive communication between scientists and journalists. For this to happen, the committee noted, science required decent leadership.

The Government responded to the Lords' endeavours by calling *Science and Society* a 'seminal report'. It signalled its commitment to 'a more open style of regulatory process' by pointing to public hearings about the risks from bovine spongiform encephalopathy and the implications of human genetics research. Government endorsed the select committee's recommendations to strengthen COPUS, to support the role of the MRC (and other research councils) in promoting public discussion of science, to study further the way in which risk is communicated to the public, and to work harder in finding ways to interest non-scientists in science. The DTI's Office of Science and Technology was to be in the vanguard of these initiatives.

On the invitation of the Science Minister, Lord Sainsbury, the British Association for the Advancement of Science submitted its advice to government about how science could be better supported in November 2002. The British Association proposed improved monitoring of scientific events and issues in society, supported by regular national surveys of public participation in and opinions about science.

The main conclusion of their work was that the Government had little systematic understanding of the range, public perception and impact of science in society. The Office of Science and Technology largely agreed with the British Association's proposals. But there were few new initiatives for government to throw its weight behind. None of this bureaucratic expansion of mapping and monitoring was especially inspiring. It was largely tinkering mixed with drudgery.

By contrast, since 2000 and outside government, Britain has seen a period of unprecedented fertility in ideas for connecting science to the public. One example of an entirely new public institution created in direct response to the House of Lords report is the Science Media Centre. The Science Media Centre exists 'to promote the voices, stories, and views of the scientific community to the news media when science is in the headlines'. It lives under the auspices of the Royal Institution.

In the Centre's inaugural report reviewing its remit and role, an even larger strategic goal was set out: 'to help renew public trust in science by working to promote more balanced, accurate and rational coverage' of controversial science subjects. The aim was to exploit media opportunities in order 'to make the case for science'. It acts as a resource for non-specialist journalists, scientists, and science press officers. The Centre describes itself as 'unashamedly pro-science'.

Even more important is what the Centre does not do. It does not seek to be a leader in matters of science and medicine. The Centre does not promote itself directly to the media. It does not offer any immediate service to the public. It does not publicize its own research. And it does not issue its own statements on matters of medical or scientific controversy. But the Centre does take sides when it deems it necessary to do so. For example, '. . . in an area of major public concern such as the MMR vaccine, where the vast majority of scientists took one view and the alternative view was held by a very tiny minority (but received disproportionate media exposure), it was important that the SMC work with the majority of scientists to help get their case across'. The Centre is aware of the risk of being seen as the Chief Spinner for UK Science. But it denies the accusation that it attempts to control the news agenda. Given that journalism is so often about controversy and conflict, the Centre only seeks 'to ensure that media coverage of controversial science issues is not imbalanced'. That difficult word again.

By contrast, Sense About Science tries to be more prominent. Founded in 2002 and chaired by Lord Dick Taverne, this charitable trust aims 'to encourage an evidence-based approach to scientific and technological developments'. Its twin concerns are public education and understanding. Taverne, a former barrister, has been a vocal critic of the Legal Aid Board funded work into the safety of the MMR vaccine. He has, for example, drawn attention to the weak scientific credentials of lawyers involved in this litigation. And he has called this entire episode of inappropriate lawyerly intrusion into what was essentially a matter for scientists to resolve a 'disgrace', a 'farce', and a 'scandal'. Unfortunately, Sense about Science has allowed itself to become an easy target for attack. Its financial donors include GlaxoSmithKline, one of the manufacturers of the MMR vaccine and a defendant in the litigation brought by claimant families. Among the forty-five people who make up Sense About Science's board of trustees and advisory council, there are Lords (five), Knights (seven), Professors (fifteen), luminous Fellows (fourteen), distinguished doctors (twelve), a Baroness and a Dame. There is only one lay representative – the cook and writer Prue Leith. There are no representatives from patient groups or mildly dissident non-governmental organizations. The waters of orthodoxy will surely remain beautifully calm: more Silence than Sense About Science.

Both the Science Media Centre and Sense About Science are based in London. But other more interesting and in many ways more creative initiatives have sprung up all around Britain. One of the most significant is the idea of the Café Scientifique. This is a forum where scientists will meet over a coffee, a drink or an informal dinner with anybody who cares to turn up. They talk about and debate issues that are both topical and of wide public interest. It may be the launch of a book (I have been fortunate enough to have taken part in Cafés Scientifiques in Leeds, Lancaster and London discussing and defending the MMR vaccine, among many other subjects) or the emergence of a particular new controversy that prompts a group to gather. Or it could simply be that an interesting person is keen to get out and discuss science (Colin Blakemore was especially active at these cafés when he took over at the Medical Research Council in 2003). There are now twenty active cafés in the UK, many of them supported by the Wellcome Trust. From the Orkney Islands to Plymouth, and from Belfast to Cardiff, they are a wonderful way to discuss and argue about science. Totally inclusive, entirely informal, and driven by curiosity and passion, there are no lecture theatres, there is no insufferable academic pomposity, and there is a welcome absence of oak-panelled institutional torpor. Just pure enthusiasm. They suggest a reincarnation of the cafés of the eighteenth-century when Enlightenment ideas began to trickle out of the scientific world and into politics, religion and the economy. Every town should have one.

The other great innovation was to treat science as one would any aspect of the arts. There is an Edinburgh Festival. So why not a Science Festival? Cheltenham has festivals for jazz, music and literature. In 2002, the city launched a Festival of Science. Held each June over five days, the festival is serious and entertaining, orthodox and wild. There are debates, talks, discussions, practical demonstrations, readings, and moments of pure whimsy – with subjects such as the science of whisky, perfume or Spiderman, and issues that have stretched from AIDS to atomic physics. The wide divide between science and entertainment is successfully bridged. Children and schools make up a central part of the programme. This remarkable mix is the essence of real engagement. The Cheltenham Festival of Science is a huge and incredible success. This *is* science *in* society.[9]

Meanwhile, the Royal Society continues to develop its relatively small programme in support of science communication, education, and public dialogue (one of its seven objectives). To these ends, the Royal Society puts scientists in schools; celebrates science with an annual Michael Faraday Award for Science Communication (the winner in 2003 was David Attenborough); orchestrates a varied programme of public lectures, exhibitions and events; and in 2001, again after taking account of the House of Lords report, embarked on a five-year science in society programme. This initiative pairs scientists with Members of Parliament in an effort to help both sides better understand each other's work, the lack of which was a source of much irritation to scientists in the past. The Royal Society also organizes regional and national consultations – for example on trust in science, genetics and health, and cybersecurity – all with the goal of bringing scientists directly into contact with the public – activities that have not led to the intractable confrontations some might have predicted.

Occasionally the Royal Society finds it hard to stop itself acting like the authoritarian parent it is trying not to be. Its *Guidelines on Science and Health Communication*, published in November 2001, were distinguished only by the speed with which they moved from the postroom to the dustbin. It is hard to imagine a moment when more condescending, although well-meaning, advice to professional journalists has ever been provided. 'Have the findings been published in a peer-reviewed journal?' intoned the Society to reporters.

(What has that got to do with news, I have heard journalists ask.) 'Do these findings appear to contradict mainstream scientific opinion?' (If they do, all the better, perhaps, from a news perspective.) 'Will the report cause undue anxiety or optimism among audiences or readers?' (A journalist is not the Chief Medical Officer.) It was as if the House of Lords report had never been published. The Royal Society's guidelines were quickly and quietly shelved. Even insiders within the Royal Society now concede that this effort at improving science communication was badly misjudged.

But in surveying the rich range of public offerings provided by people who want to see a stronger civic appreciation of science, there is one enormous gap. Leadership. No single organization cuts across these different activities, coordinating responses to controversies, initiating investigations into new concerns, or acting as a lightning rod for sudden flashes of public anxiety. This organization would need to be highly visible. It would need to have authority, but be located outside of government. It would need to be seen to operate a process that encourages participation in decision-making, and so avoid the mistake of issuing declarations from an elite of the great and the good.

When the House of Lords Select Committee discussed the issue of leadership, COPUS seemed to be one body that could take on at least part of this role. The Government agreed. In its response to the House of Lords report, it concluded that 'COPUS will almost certainly have an important role to play in encouraging Government and independent bodies to enhance their dialogue activities, and to encourage them to reach members of the general public who are not normally engaged by such activities.' Back in 2000, COPUS planned to be an umbrella body for science. It intended to broaden its membership. It would extend its network and consultative functions. It would seek full-time staff to establish its long-term future.

It would move away from the rather patronizing idea of 'public understanding' (premise: the public are ignorant) to something more collaborative, such as 'Science and the public in partnership'. Yet the outcome for COPUS has been bad. The Committee ceased to function in 2002, after a series of acrimonious exchanges between its members and the sponsoring organizations. A joint statement by the British Association, the Royal Institution and the Royal Society said, rather tersely and contrary to every opinion hitherto given, that: 'We have reached the conclusion that the top-down approach which COPUS currently exemplifies is no longer appropriate to the wider agenda that the science communication community is now addressing.'

All that remains is a vestigial funding scheme to encourage public access to science. COPUS is dead, in all but name. In the meantime, the British Association, the Royal Institution, the Royal Society, research funding bodies, museums and science centres all do their own thing. Pluralism rules, and this is largely a good thing. But a wide gap of leadership still exists nevertheless. The fact is that no single institution takes responsibility for dealing with scientific controversies when they arise. Part of this vacuum – a place where deliberations and judgements would take place about a range of scientific and medical controversies – should be filled by a National Agency on Science and Health (see Chapter 2).

Indeed, the situation for science in society seems to be deteriorating. The debate over the safety of MMR vaccination is an all too telling example of this decline into unreason. So important is this issue that the US Institute of Medicine, in its report on the alleged links between vaccines and autism, concluded that programmes should be developed to increase public participation in vaccine safety research and policy decision-making. Scientists should also improve their skills and their willingness, both largely lamentable, 'to engage in constructive dialogue with the public about research findings and their implications for policy development'. That this continues to matter is shown by the ongoing efforts of a few to promulgate concerns about the MMR vaccine. Andrew Wakefield was still speaking out about the MMR vaccine in 2004, even after the *Lancet*'s retraction. In June 2004, for example, he was advertised as talking in London about the vaccine under the headline title of 'What doctors don't tell you.'

In April 2002, Prime Minister Tony Blair gave what is widely considered to be the most important pro-science political speech of recent times. He spoke of science 'posing hard questions of moral judgement and of practical concern'. He called for 'a proper understanding of what science is trying to achieve'. And he emphasized that 'We need better, stronger, clearer ways of science and people communicating . . . to re-establish trust and confidence in the way that science can demonstrate new opportunities, and offer new solutions.'

But at the end of 2003, a completely ridiculous but nevertheless damaging controversy surfaced about the way British honours were awarded to scientists. It was suggested that Colin Blakemore, the MRC's chief executive, had been denied a knighthood because of 'his controversial work on vivisection'. Blakemore hit out with searing criticism of the Government's duplicitous approach to science, lauding it in public but denying its leading exponents honours when their work touched a highly sensitive nerve of public concern, such as animal experimentation. For a few difficult days, the Government was thrown on the defensive, as Blakemore – in his words, 'angry, upset, and embarrassed' – threatened to resign from the MRC. Ministers hastily offered their support for Blakemore's animal research, while diverting blame away from themselves and on to the civil service system that awards honours. It was a silly and ignominious moment for the Government, undoing much of its previous rhetorical commitment to science in society. What became abundantly clear was that science needed its own trusted advocates, since none would ever be reliably found in government.

Who might these advocates be? Who can occupy that rather dangerous space between the media (which acts as the only effective route to the public) and the overlapping worlds of medicine and science? Here there is nothing but a gaping hole. Science has few public intellectuals to make its case to wider society. That role seems to have been left to politicians – a grave error, as I shall show in a moment.

What do I mean by public intellectual? I mean somebody who is an expert in a particular field of study and who has the ability to communicate that expertise to a wider non-specialist audience. Public intellectuals are not high-profile journalists. They are not celebrity columnists. They have a reputation of distinction in their own academic sphere of activity. But they also have qualities that take them beyond that often narrow niche.

Who are the public intellectuals for science and medicine? In an entertaining but nevertheless telling competition run by the British magazine *Prospect* in July 2004, the beginnings of an answer emerged. And how disappointing that answer was. *Prospect* asked readers to vote for Britain's top public intellectuals. One hundred people were listed, but only nine received over one hundred votes, my threshold for identifying those who stood out from the crowd. So who were they? Richard Dawkins, Germaine Greer, Amartya Sen, Eric Hobsbawm, Jonathan Miller, Timothy Garton Ash, Simon Schama, Michael Ignatieff and Melvyn Bragg. Although Jonathan Miller was once a practising doctor, I doubt that he would lay claim to any special understanding about the safety of the MMR vaccine. And nor, I suspect, would Richard Dawkins. Which leaves . . . precisely no one. Of course, there have been commentators on the MMR vaccine who have transcended their usual academic territory. In the *London Review of Books*, Hugh Pennington, a respected microbiologist, asked 'Why can't doctors be more scientific?' in assessing the evidence about vaccines (he was particularly critical of me). And the general practitioner Michael Fitzpatrick, in his book *MMR and Autism*, presents a very detailed analysis of almost every aspect of the Wakefield affair. But neither Pennington nor Fitzpatrick has achieved the kind of awareness and authority to make a difference in the public's mind. Science and medicine need an Edward Said or a Joseph Stiglitz. We have Robert Winston and Colin Blakemore. But they work as educators or on the margins of wider public discourse. Our society needs more Winstons and Blakemores, and we need to put them centre stage in public disputes about technical matters of public anxiety.

The House of Lords let journalists off lightly. And, so far, so have I. Yet I began this chapter by indicating that journalism is passing through a period as uncomfortable, if not more so, as that for science and medicine. This state of affairs is proven annually in a survey of over 2,000 adults aged fifteen years or over in Great Britain. The MORI poll is conducted on behalf of the British Medical Association. When people were asked in 2004 whether they generally trusted those in the following occupations to tell the truth, they replied:

Occupation	Tell the truth (%)	Not tell the truth (%)	Don't know (%)
Doctors	92	5	3
Teachers	89	7	5

Professors	80	9	11
Judges	75	16	8
Scientists	69	19	12
Civil Servants	51	37	13
Business leaders	30	58	13
Government ministers	23	70	8
Politicians generally	22	71	7
Journalists	20	72	8

The British Medical Association uses these figures to bolster the public reputation of doctors. One could easily use them to discredit the reputations of journalists. Criticism of journalists from within government is especially strong. Geoff Mulgan, who worked as head of policy in 10 Downing Street until 2004, has called attention to an 'ethical deficit at the core of the information society'.[10] He criticized what he saw as the absence of a moral compass – 'a strong ethic of searching for the truth' – in the media. The consequence was that, for many journalists, the truth of what they print seems irrelevant to the larger good of selling newspapers. 'The net result,' Mulgan wrote, 'is that the public are left with systematically incorrect perspectives on the world.' Doctors have made similar remarks about the media.[11]

It is worth adding a parenthesis here. The MORI data show that government ministers are trusted only marginally more than journalists. But here there is a paradox in the MMR vaccine story. In the research that the UK Department of Health has conducted on public views about diseases and vaccines, government scientists have come to the view that the public wants clear, consistent and factual information from government about immunization. Given this attitude, between 2001 and 2003 the Department of Health distributed 160,000 MMR vaccine information packs for parents, sent 624,000 leaflets to general practices, put up 31,000 posters, produced 50,000 videos and created a website devoted entirely to the MMR vaccine. This work was a formidable public relations exercise. But the MORI poll results indicate that little of this information will have been trusted.

The House of Lords report did gently raise matters that it wished journalists would attend to. The select committee urged a more nuanced understanding of uncertainty, a more sophisticated treatment of risk, and a greater appreciation of journalistic responsibility. But journalists counter that these injunctions do a disservice to the intelligence of their readers. As the *Guardian*'s science editor, Tim Radford, put it in 1996 in the *Lancet*:[12]

> The public shows a remarkable capacity to enjoy the cavalcade of hypocritical, frivolous or malicious entertainments served up for it. It also shows a remarkable ability to distinguish the stuff that does matter from the stuff that does not, and a comforting capacity to be confused when the situation is genuinely confusing. The readership of a newspaper seems to behave remarkably like any sensible individual: perfectly happy to be entertained, mostly capable of discerning important patterns in the flood of competing signals, and unlikely to be misled about the things that really will alter his or her life, or their way of looking at it.

Until, one might add, Andrew Wakefield came along. In the context of the friction surrounding the MMR vaccine, what many journalists – and their editors – have failed to realize is the incredible power they sometimes hold over the public's attitudes. The UK Department of Health has found, for example, that parents' decisions to delay or refuse the MMR vaccine correlate closely with the newspaper they read, and so the editorial line that the newspaper adopts about the vaccine's safety. So why did it all go so wrong with Wakefield?

In *Risk and Reason*,[13] the American legal scholar Cass Sunstein examines how unjustified fears have come to be one of the most serious challenges facing the governance of modern democratic societies. Anxieties develop, Sunstein argues, because they are too easily allowed to develop. When a signal of risk is proposed, each one of us confirms or refutes that risk individually by searching for examples from our own experience. If a personal example is available to us to draw on, it will tend to support our own suspicion about the genuine existence of that risk. By telling others of our experience and the connection we have made between that experience and the risk, we trigger an 'availability cascade' – a chain of response that propagates a fear, increasing its availability still further to others until a mass delusion is established. These informal and often scientifically uninformed networks and cascades are a profound source of worry to public health workers. The media usually widens these networks and amplifies these cascades by increasing the pool of personal examples each one of us can draw on. The result is a gross public over estimation of any given risk.

The media does something more. It can frame the risk in such a way as to create vivid mental pictures that drive a demand for government regulation. Common affective triggers include extreme human suffering, the involvement of vulnerable groups in society (for example, children), and risks that we have no or little control over. If people believe that an activity is dangerous, they tend to believe it has few benefits. But if one is aware that a technology has a high, visible and demonstrable advantage, small risks are easily put into their proper context and accommodated. Scares about the health effects of mobile telephones, for example, had zero impact on long-term mobile telephone use – mobile phones were too obviously useful for anybody to take such poorly substantiated claims seriously. The lesson, perhaps, is that as a society we need to find better ways to strengthen our cultural memory by repeatedly reminding ourselves of the advances and benefits that we now take for granted. For the MMR vaccine, that means recalling the untrammelled human effects of measles. When parents have no fear of the disease, their likely and completely understandable response will be to refuse the vaccine (if they are anxious about its safety) or to ignore it (if they are not).

These issues have not been lost on journalists.[14] Matters of ethics, truth and values are now a regular subject for internal journalistic debate. The emergence of this meta-journalism points to a growing insecurity in the media's attitude to itself. The lack of trust that so many among the public have in journalists reflects a cancer on the body of news, one that has metastasized with unusual aggression to the science and health desks. Ian Hargreaves, a former editor of the *Independent* and the *New Statesman*, restates the standard view that 'the first job of journalism is to find out, communicate accurately, and be trusted'. This statement of purpose is his response to the present widespread criticism of the press.

But such a platitude ignores the vast range of journalistic styles one will encounter in a newsroom. Richard Keeble, in his *Ethics for Journalists*, anatomizes these styles as cynicism (profits are the root of all journalism so why bother with such idealistic fancies as ethics?), professionalism (a 'commitment to journalistic standards'), and individual conscience ('ethical relativism'). Still, in the context of science and medicine, none of these approaches takes us very far.

The best analysis of journalism today that I know of comes from the Pulitzer Prize winning writer and a publisher of the *Chicago Tribune*, Jack Fuller. He calls, contrary to the wishes of scientists and politicians, for a much more critical relationship between journalists and science. In *News Values*, Fuller writes that

Journalism is supposed to illuminate matters of public concern, and this includes the job of discovering significant information that otherwise might be hidden. So journalism *must* approach science . . . with the same disciplined scepticism with which it approaches the activities of a city council or a governor.

To do this job effectively, journalists need to be well-versed in contemporary science and medicine, perhaps with a specialized degree in the subject they are covering. Here is Jack Fuller again: 'Since most journalists are never taught to read an article in a scientific journal critically, is it any wonder that they report flawed research as definitive and narrow conclusions as sweeping?'

The exemplar of this view was Victor Cohn, a former science editor for the *Washington Post*. His book, *News and Numbers: a Guide to Reporting Statistical Claims and Controversies in Health and Other Stories,* will be found in almost every serious newsroom and is a standard reference work at American journalism schools.[15] Britain needs a Victor Cohn. That is, a journalist who works in science and medical news every day of their working lives and who will wave the flag for critical but knowledgeable scrutiny of research. Only a very few of our present health and science correspondents match up to the Cohn standard. The story of Andrew Wakefield and the MMR vaccine sadly attests to the truth of this view. It is one of the greatest flaws in British journalism today.

Of course, one could justifiably argue that medical journal editors should do more to dampen down the potentially damaging controversies that they ignite. Victor Cohn put it like this:

I believe that in a day when the reports in medical and other journals are widely scanned by TV and print reporters and conveyed to the public – not to mention scanned by highly non-statistical physicians, bless them – editors should take into account that, intentionally or not, they are now reporting to the public and to patients. This should mean including – it need only be very brief – the context that the public as well as physicians who talk to their patients need. It means answering the unanswered questions.

Cohn was right. This should be an urgent priority for all editors of scientific and medical journals. Medical journal editors – and, indeed, the public – must also be more conscious of the part peer-review can play in testing new ideas before publication. Yet peer-review is not a perfect tool. It is not a single event that is performed once in the lifetime of an idea. Peer-review is a continuous process of criticism and inquiry, beginning from the very first moment a new concept is originated and lasting to the time when that idea is discarded, accepted or modified into a better approximation of how we understand the world. Wakefield's work was unusual in that it crossed the borders of many medical specialties – psychiatry, neurology, gastroenterology, paediatrics, virology, communicable disease, vaccines and public health. This kind of multidisciplinary research can put extreme strain on even the best and most rigorous system of peer-review.

I am also keenly aware that the *Lancet* has been criticized for giving Wakefield a platform to defend himself even after his 1998 paper was published – and heavily attacked. Given the ferocity with which he was targeted, I can hardly see – on simple grounds of fairness – how we could have done otherwise. But I recognize that his pariah status revoked, for some at least, his right to be heard in the pages of a scientific journal. I have also been told by senior Department of Health officials that we should have published more of the research that refuted Wakefield's hypothesis. In fact, we quickly published three studies rejecting his claims. We also turned away several more studies objecting to his identification of the MMR vaccine as a potential cause of autism – all after thorough peer-review. Our critics cannot have it both ways. They want tough peer-review, but they sometimes seem to want its consequences to work only in one direction – against Wakefield. This is not peer-review. It is peer-bias.

Indeed, despite these uncomfortable events, medical journal editors must not refrain from publishing work that challenges mainstream scientific, clinical or public health opinion. There are now strong forces operating on journals to protect the system of health messages distributed to the public. The media is so voracious in its appetite for controversy, it is so merciless in its challenges to conventional opinion, that medical journals should, so many doctors will argue, avoid fuelling these fires. Journal editors should try to keep these difficult discussions within a closed professional circle. I simply do not accept this argument. It is a recipe for the stagnation of knowledge and the creation of a wholly undemocratic technocracy. If there is a weakness in the evidential basis for any drug, device or vaccine, then we should be honest and open enough to say so. We should work to remove that weakness. Better still, we should have done the research to avoid that weakness in the first place. Secrecy leads to complacency, complacency to avoidable error.

What role therefore, does the press have in protecting the public from scares based on weak evidence? The press is usually considered to be a watchdog over the state. This role, so the orthodoxy goes, overrides all others. But who watches the watchdog? In the UK and for newspapers, it is the Press Complaints Commission. Many doctors and scientists I know consider that, when it comes to accuracy and balance (balance as defined by scientists, not journalists), voluntary self-regulation by the media is nowhere nearly sufficient to do this job properly. I do not want to see greater regulation of press coverage of science and medicine, and certainly not as a response to the MMR vaccine episode. Bad cases make bad law. Further regulation and new penalties will only diminish the motivation for critical scrutiny of science – a poor outcome for the public. But a system that monitors and reports on press accuracy would be a valuable step forward. We all do our jobs better if we know that someone, somewhere is evaluating what we do.

Geoff Mulgan has suggested that the universities could do this work. They might, he wrote, 'play a more active role in assuring standards, investigating errors, and holding to account journalists and media outlets against an ethic of truth and accuracy'. I think this is a useful idea to pursue. It is one that could easily be taken up by an enterprising academic journalism department. Such oversight is common in the US – look at the excellent *Columbia Journalism Review* – but it is largely dismissed in Britain as taking the media far too seriously. Whereas in the US journalism falls within the realm of erudite political science, in the UK it leans more towards savage literary criticism. If universities are not willing to take up the challenge, I would create a new role of media ombudsman within NASH. His or her job would be to observe, describe, investigate and report on how the media cover science and medicine. A media ombudsman for science and medicine would act as a curb on exaggerated interpretations of controversial research.[16]

I have tried to sketch out some of the wider lessons that we collectively might learn from the events surrounding publication of Andrew Wakefield's work in the *Lancet*, together with his subsequent investigations and claims. Domestically, I have argued that we must rethink the institutional arrangements that govern the democratic control of science in society. Specifically, I have proposed two new institutions to meet the greater demand for independent scrutiny of scientific controversies and of science itself – a National Agency for Science and Health and a Council for Research Integrity. I have also tried to make the case for scaling up investment into autism care and research to meet a large and hidden need in society. I have raised concern that the science community, in particular its leadership, has failed to meet the challenges set out by the landmark 2000 House of Lords Select Committee report. I have also criticized the increasing commercialization of scientific research and the way in which so many scientists seem to have sold their souls at the altar of wealth creation, led and endorsed by a narrow governmental interpretation of science as little more than an extension of the Department of Trade and Industry.

Finally, I have tried to underline the present-day weaknesses in science and health journalism, and in the way that health research is described and interpreted on the internet and in the growing number of self-help books written for the public. Many of these lessons are not confined to Britain alone. But globally, the one area that truly should concern us is the burden of measles infection in the most disadvantaged nations of the world. The next few years will be critical for laying down the strategies and techniques for eradicating this entirely preventable infection that needlessly kills over half a million people, mostly children, every year.

Is it unreasonable to believe that one day we might live in problem-solving civic communities that, if confronted by a signal of concern, seek to be informed by scientific evidence and governed by rational procedures of deliberation and decision-making? As violence becomes the dominant diplomatic language in the opening years of a new century, this restatement of such a fundamental Enlightenment principle might seem strangely quaint and outmoded for today's world. Yet if we accept Stuart Hampshire's argument that justice is indeed (and inherently) conflict, and that managing this conflict with the right set of institutions and procedures is the best means we have at our disposal to create the conditions for justice, then our flourishing media cyberculture, together with the rapid enfranchisement of millions of new voices within that culture, offers possibilities for a mosaic of conversations that might come close to Hampshire's – if not my – ideal.

As Niccolò Machiavelli once realized, in his remarkable study of state politics in the sixteenth century,[17] deception is best overcome by immersing oneself in the detail of the question at hand. 'It is clear that the quickest way to open the people's eyes,' he wrote, 'given that a general matter may deceive them, is to make them get down to its particulars.' We eliminate error, overcome weak evidence, and refute false arguments best of all in a thriving culture of debate, dissent, and criticism. This is as true in the public sphere as it is in the scientific sphere.

In an ever-intensifying network of impersonal expert systems that regulate our lives today, our survival – resting as it does on our continued confidence and trust in those systems – depends on our shared belief in the unrestrained freedom of others to contradict and disprove our opinions. No matter how strenuously we hold a particular point of view, this common bond of engagement is our safeguard in preventing passion from descending into tyranny and reason from mutating into arrogance. This is the final lesson to be learned from the debate over the safety of the MMR vaccine.

Is it impossible to suppose that, after an alarming detour into the catacombs of irrationalism, this upheaval might have strengthened the culture of science in society? Certainly, I believe that it has reinforced our desire for rational decision-making in public life. And that it has reiterated the need to strip away the mystique from science, throwing open its doors fully to public scrutiny. For only by doing so will we avoid a dystopia of Atwoodian proportions.

APPENDIX

The full report of the allegations made in February 2004 against the authors of the 1998 *Lancet* paper, together with rebuttal statements by Dr Wakefield, Dr Murch, Professor Walker-Smith, and the Royal Free Hospital, was published in the *Lancet* on 6 March 2004. A summary of the journal's findings is reported here in full.

A STATEMENT BY THE EDITORS OF *THE LANCET*

On February 18, 2004, serious allegations of research misconduct concerning an article by Dr Andrew Wakefield and colleagues published in *The Lancet* in February, 1998,[1] were brought to the attention of senior editorial staff of the journal.

The allegations are:

(1) That, contrary to a statement in the *Lancet* paper, ethics approval for the investigations conducted on the children reported in the study, some of them highly invasive (eg, lumbar puncture), had not been given.

(2) That the study reported in *The Lancet* was completed under the cover of ethics approval for an entirely different study of 25 children with 'A new paediatric syndrome: enteritis and disintegrative disorder following measles/rubella vaccination'.

(3) That, contrary to the statement in the *Lancet* paper that children were 'consecutively referred to the department of paediatric gastroenterology' at the Royal Free Hospital and School of Medicine, children were invited to participate in the study by Dr Andrew Wakefield and Professor John Walker-Smith, thus biasing the selection of children in favour of families reporting an association between their child's illness and the MMR vaccine.

(4) That the children who were reported in the *Lancet* study were also part of a Legal Aid Board funded pilot project, led by Dr Wakefield – a pilot project with the aim of investigating the grounds for pursuing a multi-party legal action on behalf of parents of allegedly vaccine-damaged children, the existence of which was not disclosed to the editors of *The Lancet.*

(5) That the results eventually reported in the 1998 *Lancet* paper were passed to lawyers and used to justify the multi-party legal action prior to publication, a fact that was not disclosed to the editors of *The Lancet.*

(6) That Dr Wakefield received £55,000 from the Legal Aid Board to conduct this pilot project and that, since there was a substantial overlap of children in both the Legal Aid Board funded pilot project and the *Lancet* paper, this was a financial conflict of interest that should have been declared to the editors and was not.[2]

The editors of *The Lancet* have seen and reviewed the documentary evidence available in support of these allegations. In acting on this information we have followed the guidelines on dealing with alleged misconduct as set out by the UK Committee on

Publication Ethics, on which representatives of *The Lancet* sit. We have presented this evidence to the senior authors of the 1998 *Lancet* paper (Dr Wakefield, Professor John Walker-Smith, Dr Peter Harvey, and Dr Simon Murch) in order to seek their responses. Dr Richard Horton, Editor of *The Lancet*, has also shared this information with Professor Humphrey Hodgson, vice-Dean and campus director of the Royal Free and University College Medical School, London, the institution at which the original work took place.

With this notice are accompanying statements from Dr Murch, Professor Walker-Smith, and Dr Wakefield, answering the allegations of research and publication misconduct, together with a statement from the Royal Free and University College Medical School.

Given these four statements, together with an evaluation of the available documents, we consider that:

Allegation 1

The evidence we have seen indicates that ethics committee approval was given for data collection from clinically indicated investigations in the children with an initially undiagnosed illness and who were described in the 1998 *Lancet* paper. This illness was at first believed to be enteritis combined with a disintegrative disorder. Subsequent detailed clinical investigations eventually showed this condition to be the syndrome finally reported in *The Lancet*. This course of events was not described in full in the *Lancet* paper, although the similarity of the behavioural changes with those of a disintegrative psychosis (Heller's disease) were commented on in the discussion section of the 1998 *Lancet* paper. In summary, the evidence does not support this allegation.

Allegation 2

As described under Allegation 1, detailed clinically appropriate investigations led to a re-evaluation of the initial diagnosis of these children, as set out in protocol 172-96. The evidence we have seen indicates that there was no attempt by investigators to conduct the study of children reported in *The Lancet* in 1998 under cover of an entirely different investigation. In sum, the evidence does not support this allegation.

Allegation 3

Professor Walker-Smith notes that although the referral pattern was unusual – direct contact by patients with Dr Wakefield leading to referral to the Royal Free – the children were indeed consecutively referred. He reports that to the best of his recollection he did not invite any children to participate in the study. Thus, as far as the facts can be ascertained by a review of the case notes and from memory, children reported in the 1998 *Lancet* paper were consecutively referred to the Royal Free and were not deliberately sought by the authors for inclusion in their study based on parents' beliefs about an association between their child's illness and the MMR vaccine.

Allegations 4–6

Dr Wakefield had two roles in this work. First, he was the lead investigator of a Royal Free study into the nature of a new syndrome with bowel and psychiatric symptoms. Second, he was commissioned through a lawyer to undertake virological investigations as part of a study funded by the Legal Aid Board. At the time of submission and eventual publication of his 1998 *Lancet* paper, this second study had not been disclosed to the editors of *The Lancet*. We judge that it should have been so disclosed, irrespective of the number of children overlapping between the pilot project funded by the Legal Aid Board and the *Lancet* paper. Such a disclosure would have provided important information to editors and peer reviewers about the context in which this work was taking place – a context that would have been vital in making a final decision about publication. We believe that our conflict of interest guidelines at the time should have triggered such a disclosure, including the fact that a significant minority of the children described in the *Lancet* paper were also part of the Legal Aid Board funded pilot project. These guidelines stated that: 'The conflict of interest test is a simple one. Is there anything . . . that would embarrass you if it were to emerge after publication and you had not declared it?'

The difficulty of adopting a dual role as a clinical investigator and as a participant in an evaluation on behalf of the Legal Aid Board is revealed in Dr Wakefield's response to Allegation 5. Although it may be correct that 'this [*Lancet*] publication . . . added nothing further to the issue of causation than that that was already well known to the lawyers', the perception of a potential conflict of interest remains. Editors and reviewers should have had an opportunity to take his dual role into consideration when assessing this paper for publication.

Finally, although the Legal Aid Board funding referred to a different aspect of Dr Wakefield's work from that reported in *The Lancet*, the perception of a conflict of interest nevertheless remains. This funding source should, we judge, have been disclosed to the editors of the journal.

Summary

The first three allegations of alleged research misconduct have been answered by clarifications provided by the senior authors of this work. The wording in the published paper regarding Ethical Practice Committee approval and patient referral was accurate, yet at the same time summarized obviously lengthy and complex institutional and clinical review and referral procedures. In the light of the public controversy surrounding this work and the allegations made to us, one could argue that more explanation could and should have been provided in the original paper. Although, with hindsight, this seems a reasonable criticism, all research papers published by all journals are inevitably concise accounts of often complicated research protocols. We do not judge that there was any intention to conceal information or deceive editors, reviewers, or readers about the ethical justification for this work and the nature of patient referral. We are pleased to have had the opportunity to clarify the scientific record over the matters raised by these serious allegations.

We regret that aspects of funding for parallel and related work and the existence of ongoing litigation that had been known during clinical evaluation of the children reported in the 1998 *Lancet* paper were not disclosed to editors. We also regret that the overlap between children in the *Lancet* paper and in the Legal Aid Board funded pilot project was not revealed to us. We judge that all this information would have been material to our decision-making about the paper's suitability, credibility, and validity for publication.

In considering what sanctions *The Lancet* should apply, the COPE guidelines[3] give eight options in a ranked order of severity. Given the public-health importance of MMR vaccination, together with the public interest in this issue, we have decided to pursue a course of full disclosure and transparency concerning these allegations, the authors' responses, the institution's judgement, and our evaluation.

Richard Horton

Simon Murch went on to 'refute the allegation' concerning lack of ethics committee approval 'absolutely'. John Walker-Smith denied the claim that there was 'systematic bias in the pattern of referral for the children'. The Royal Free Hospital, in the guise of Professor Humphrey Hodgson, its taciturn vice-dean, commented that research conducted by Wakefield and his collaborators 'had been subjected to appropriate and rigorous ethical scrutiny'.

The statement we published by Andrew Wakefield was the most poignant of all. It seemed to reflect the state of mind of a man brought close to ruin by events to which he knew he had contributed substantially. There was a sense of defeat in what he had to say, a feeling of weariness and resignation as the battle he had started so long ago now entered its final phase. He wrote:

> The clinical and pathological findings in these children stand as reported . . . I regret the difficulties that this issue has caused my colleagues over the last week and I am grateful to them for their advice and support . . . My colleagues and I have acted at all times in the best medical interests of these children and will continue to do so.

I could not help but feel that these were the words of a good man brought low by an exceptional mélange of personality traits. Some saw these traits as desperate failings. But such a conviction, while resonant with the medical zeitgeist, seems to me unfair. Wakefield was hasty and at times ill-considered in his actions. He did let his desire to be an advocate for these children – a perfectly reasonable role to adopt in ordinary circumstances – cloud his scientific judgement when he advocated splitting the MMR vaccine at the Royal Free Hospital's press conference in 1998. But these were not, and never had been, ordinary circumstances. He had lit the fuse of a gunpowder trail that could not be extinguished. His pride had made it impossible for him to retreat honourably from an extreme and ultimately untenable position.

But these character traits did not make him a poor doctor, let alone a bad man. He did make mistakes in the way that he acted – sometimes foolish, sometimes grave mistakes. He should have disclosed his potential conflict of interest; he should not have advocated splitting the MMR vaccine into its component elements in such a public and unqualified way; he did refuse to take part in the partial retraction of his paper when invited to do so by those well placed to advise him.

Wakefield was guilty of naïveté, of relying on flawed intuition, of equating instinct with evidence, and of allowing his beliefs to drive a series of public statements that cracked the foundation stone of one of Britain's most important programmes for protecting the health of its children. For some people, these were irresponsible acts that could never be forgiven. For others, myself included, they threw into sharp relief more systemic failings of a medical and public health system that was and remains poorly designed to meet the needs of today's more questioning, sceptical, and inquiring public.[4]

NOTES

INTRODUCTION

1 See Andrew Wakefield and colleagues, 'Ileal-lymphoid-nodular hyperplasia, non-specific colitis, and pervasive developmental disorder in children', *Lancet* 1998; 351: 637–42.

2 There were also some wonderful flights of fancy in all the public speculation about Wakefield and the *Lancet*. Carole Caplin, Cherie Blair's personal adviser and confidante, weighed in, claiming that 'extremely powerful forces would like nothing better than to suppress public debate'. If only that were so! Public debate seemed the one thing that we were not short of. *Private Eye* suggested that Brian Deer was likely to be engaged in a 'petulant temper tantrum' over his allegations, which I had denied, that the *Lancet* had broken a promise not to make a public statement about the evidence he had presented to us before his own article appeared in the *Sunday Times*. Jasper Gerard took up this theme in his *Sunday Times* column, accusing me of a 'sly leaking of the scandal'. For what is likely to be the only occasion in my life, he linked me to the Prime Minister: 'Blair, Horton, and this poisonous episode make me sick. What we really need is vaccinations against them.'

3 See Linqi Zhang and colleagues, 'Retraction of an interpretation', *Science* 2004; 303: 467.

4 See Matt Nixson, 'I will sue, says MMR doctor', *Mail on Sunday*, 29 February 2004, 25.

5 See Andrew Wakefield and colleagues, 'MMR – responding to retraction', *Lancet* 2004; 363: 1327–28.

CHAPTER 1: IS THE MMR VACCINE SAFE?

1 See John F. Enders, 'Francis Home and his experimental approach to medicine', *Bulletin of the History of Medicine* 1964; 38: 101–12.

2 See Peter Ludwig Panum, 'Observations made during the epidemic of measles on the Faroe Islands in the year 1846', *Medical Classics* 1939; 3: 829–86.

3 See John F. Enders and Thomas C. Peebles, 'Propagation in tissue cultures of cytopathogenic agents from patients with measles', *Proceedings of the Society for Experimental Biology and Medicine* 1954; 86: 277–86.

4 The exceptions are parental refusal and clinical contraindications, such as an impaired immune response, untreated cancer, children who have received another live vaccine by injection within the past three weeks, children with allergies to gelatin or neomycin, and children with an acute febrile illness. A personal or family history of seizures is not a contraindication. The issue of febrile seizures remains especially vexed. Febrile seizures are convulsions that occur in children who have a fever but no other observable cause for their seizure. The frequency of febrile seizures increases after the MMR vaccine, but the risks, causes, and long-term consequences are poorly understood. Any type of seizure remains a particular reason for anxiety, and understandably so, among parents. In one remarkably complete study of all children born in Denmark between 1991 and 1998, these issues were addressed in some detail. It was found that the MMR vaccine does temporarily increase the risk of febrile seizures (an extra 1-2 cases per 1,000 children vaccinated), but this risk falls back to normal after about two weeks. There were no reliably determined risk factors for developing febrile seizures after the MMR vaccine, other than a previous history of febrile seizures. Moreover, although children who had febrile seizures after MMR vaccination had a 'slightly increased rate' of further febrile seizures, there was, importantly, no long-term increased risk of epilepsy. See Mogens Vestergaard and colleagues, 'MMR vaccination and febrile seizures', *JAMA* 2004; 292: 351–7. If parents have any concerns about whether their children do have a reason not to receive the MMR vaccine, they should certainly consult their doctor.

5 For a comprehensive review see Lauri E. Markowitz and Samuel L. Katz, 'Measles Vaccine', in *Vaccines*, edited by Stanley A. Plotkin and

Edward A. Mortimer, Saunders, 1994, pp. 229–76. See also Anton J. F. Schwartz and colleagues, 'Clinical evaluation of a new measles–mumps–rubella trivalent vaccine', *American Journal of Diseases of Children* 1975; 129: 1408–12; Timo Vesikari and colleagues, 'Clinical trial of a new trivalent measles–mumps–rubella vaccine in young children', *American Journal of Diseases of Children* 1984; 138: 843–7; and Heikki Peltola and Olli Heinonen, 'Frequency of the adverse reactions to measles–mumps–rubella vaccine', *Lancet* 1986; i: 939–42.

6 See M. L. Forman and J. D. Cherry, 'Isolation of measles virus from the CSF of a child with encephalitis following measles vaccination' (abstract 13). Presented at the 77th Annual Meeting of the American Paediatric Society, 26–9 April 1967.

7 See http://www.mmrthefacts.nhs.uk/library/whatinfo.php

8 Vesikari and colleagues, 'Clinical trial'.

9 See Andrew J. Wakefield and colleagues, 'Pathogenesis of Crohn's disease: multifocal gastrointestinal infarction', *Lancet* 1989; ii: 1059–62.

10 See Andrew J. Wakefield and colleagues, 'Evidence of persistent measles virus infection in Crohn's disease', *Journal of Medical Virology* 1993; 39: 345–53; and J. Lewin and colleagues, 'Persistent measles virus infection of the intestine: confirmation by immunogold electron microscopy', *Gut* 1995; 36: 564–9.

11 See Anders Ekbom and colleagues, 'Perinatal measles infection and subsequent Crohn's disease', *Lancet* 1994; 344: 508–10.

12 See N. P. Thompson and colleagues, 'Is measles vaccination a risk factor for inflammatory bowel disease?', *Lancet* 1995; 345: 1071–4.

13 See A. J. Wakefield and colleagues, 'Ileal-lymphoid-nodular hyperplasia, non-specific colitis, and pervasive developmental disorder in children', *Lancet* 1998; 351: 637–41.

14 See Robert T. Chen and Frank DeStefano, 'Vaccine adverse events: causal or coincidental', *Lancet* 1998; 351: 611–12.

15 See Eric Fombonne, 'Inflammatory bowel disease and autism', *Lancet* 1998; 351: 955; and Heikki Peltola and colleagues, 'No evidence for measles, mumps, and rubella vaccine-associated inflammatory bowel disease or autism in a 14-year prospective study', *Lancet* 1998; 351: 1327–8.

16 See Brent Taylor and colleagues, 'Autism and measles, mumps, and

rubella vaccine: no epidemiological evidence for a causal association', *Lancet* 1999; 353: 2026–9.

17 See James A. Kaye and colleagues, 'MMR vaccine and the incidence of autism recorded by general practitioners: a time trend analysis', *BMJ* 2001; 322: 460–63; Loring Dales and colleagues, 'Time trends in autism and in MMR immunisation coverage in California', *JAMA* 2001; 285: 1183–5; Brent Taylor and colleagues, 'MMR vaccination and bowel problems or developmental regression in children with autism: population study', *BMJ* 2002; 324: 393–6; Annamari Makela and colleagues, 'Neurologic disorders after MMR vaccination', *Pediatrics* 2002; 110: 957–63; Kreesten Meldgaard Madsen and colleagues, 'A population-based study of MMR vaccination and autism', *New England Journal of Medicine* 2002; 347: 1477–82; Frank DeStefano and colleagues, 'Age at first MMR vaccination in children with autism and school-matched control subjects', *Pediatrics* 2004; 113: 259–66; and Liam Smeeth and colleagues, 'MMR vaccination and pervasive developmental disorders: a case-control study and systematic review', *Lancet* (in press).

18 See N. Andrews and colleagues, 'Recall bias, MMR, and autism', *Archives of Disease in Childhood* 2002; 87: 493–4; and R. Lingam and colleagues, 'Prevalence of autism and parentally reported triggers in a north east London population', *Archives of Disease in Childhood* 2003; 88: 666–70.

19 See Hisashri Kawashima and colleagues, 'Detection and sequencing of measles virus from peripheral mononuclear cells from patients with inflammatory bowel disease and autism', *Digestive Diseases and Sciences* 2000; 45: 723–7; Vijendra K. Singh and colleagues, 'Abnormal measles–mumps–rubella antibodies and CNS autoimmunity in children with autism', *Journal of Biomedical Science* 2002; 9: 359–64; and Vijendra K. Singh and Ryan L. Jensen, 'Elevated levels of measles antibodies in children with autism', *Pediatric Neurology* 2003; 28: 292–4.

20 Abnormal immune responses in children with autism have indeed been reported. See Harumi Jyonouchi and colleagues, 'Proinflammatory and regulatory cytokine production associated with innate and adaptive immune responses in children with autism spectrum disorders and developmental regression', *Journal of Neuroimmunology* 2001; 120: 170–79.

21 See Danielle L. Morris and colleagues, 'Measles vaccination and inflammatory bowel disease', *American Journal of Gastroenterology* 2000; 95: 3507–12.

22 See Karoly Horvath and colleagues, 'Gastrointestinal abnormalities in children with autistic disorder', *Journal of Pediatrics* 1999; 135: 559–63; A. J. Wakefield and colleagues, 'Enterocolitis in children with developmental disorders', *American Journal of Gastroenterology* 2000; 95: 2285–95; and Raoul I. Furlano and colleagues, 'Colonic CD8 and γδ T-cell infiltration with epithelial damage in children with autism', *Journal of Pediatrics* 2001; 138: 366–72.

23 See *MRC Review of Autism Research: Epidemiology and Causes*, London, Medical Research Council, December 2001.

24 See Sydney M. Finegold and colleagues, 'Gastrointestinal microflora studies in late-onset autism', *Clinical Infectious Diseases* 2002; 35 (Suppl. 1): S6–16; V. Uhlmann and colleagues, 'Potential viral pathogenic mechanism for new variant inflammatory bowel disease', *Journal of Clinical Pathology Molecular Pathology* 2002; 55: 84–90; F. Torrente and colleagues, 'Small intestinal enteropathy with epithelial IgG and complement deposition in children with regressive autism', *Molecular Psychiatry* 2002; 7: 375–82; Magee L. DeFelice and colleagues, 'Intestinal cytokines in children with pervasive developmental disorders', *American Journal of Gastroenterology* 2003; 98: 1777–82; Paul Ashwood and colleagues, 'Intestinal lymphocyte populations in children with regressive autism: evidence for extensive mucosal immunopathology', *Journal of Clinical Immunology* 2003; 23: 504–17; and Franco Torrente and colleagues, 'Focal-enhanced gastritis in regressive autism with features distinct from Crohn's and *Helicobacter pylori* gastritis', *American Journal of Gastroenterology* 2004; 99: 598–605.

25 See James Meikle, 'Alarm as mumps cases increase', *Guardian*, 27 March 2004, 7. In May 2004 the Department of Health recommended that students should be offered the MMR vaccine after a group attending a sports event in Spain became infected with mumps. Although this advice was not prompted by a Wakefield-induced decline in MMR vaccine uptake (the real reason was the failure to give children two doses of the vaccine before 1996), the Government used this episode to argue that 'these outbreaks illustrate why it is important for children to be fully vaccinated in childhood'.

26 Some critics of the MMR vaccine might argue, for example, that it is mainstream opinion and uncontroversial to argue that vaccines have been linked with chronic human diseases, although those links are much disputed. See, for example, David C. Wraith and colleagues, 'Vaccination and autoimmune disease: what is the evidence?', *Lancet* 2003; 362: 1659–66. These speculative and sometimes enticing hypotheses have little evidence in their favour. The connection between immunization (including the MMR vaccine) and a particular type (Type 1) of diabetes, for example, has been convincingly disproven. See Anders Hviid and colleagues, 'Childhood Vaccination and Type 1 Diabetes', *New England Journal of Medicine* 2004; 350: 1398–1404.

27 One notably independent source of information is the Consumers' Association. Its *Drugs and Therapeutics Bulletin* concluded in April 2003 that

> Immunization with the combined measles, mumps, and rubella (MMR) vaccine gives highly effective protection against all three diseases, and has the potential to eliminate these infections, including congenital rubella syndrome, saving many lives and preventing serious illness. In our view, there is no convincing evidence that MMR vaccine causes, or facilitates development of, either inflammatory bowel disease or autism. Similarly, we believe that there is no good reason to adopt an alternative immunization policy that allows substitution of single-antigen vaccines for the combined vaccine. Such an arrangement has no sound scientific basis and is likely to result in increased rates of disease and an attendant increase in morbidity, mortality, and risk to others. The weight of published evidence argues overwhelmingly in favour of MMR vaccine as the most effective and safest way of protecting children from measles, mumps, and rubella.

This same advice was given in the Consumers' Association's *Which?* magazine in January 2004.

28 For Wakefield's response to the recent criticisms levelled against his original 1998 *Lancet* paper, see 'Responding to retraction', *Lancet* 2004; 363: 1327–8.

29 See Tom Jefferson and colleagues, 'Unintended events following

immunization with MMR: a systematic review', *Vaccine* 2003; 21: 3954–60; and Tom Jefferson, 'Informed choice and balance are victims of the MMR–autism saga', *Lancet Infectious Diseases* 2004; 4: 135–6. Wakefield has used Jefferson's work as a means to defend his own views about the lack of safety data concerning the MMR vaccine. Jefferson has hit back at Wakefield, accusing him of misquotation. In May 2004 Jefferson wrote:

> Selective quotation and communication of results, poor methods, exaggeration of the effect of rare or benign diseases, hidden agendas, and undeclared conflicts of interest and pressure by public or private bodies render decision-making in vaccines increasingly irrational. We believe that independent research to shed impartial light on the public-health effects of vaccines (effectiveness, safety and acceptability) is absolutely essential. We believe that one way of achieving this aim is to prepare and maintain a library of single studies and systematic reviews on human vaccines. Impartially assessed and summarized evidence with a synopsis for consumers would then be available to all users for each vaccine.

See Tom Jefferson and colleagues, 'Selective quotation of evidence in vaccines research', *Lancet* 2004; 363: 1738.

30 See Michael Kidd and colleagues, 'Measles-associated encephalitis in children with renal transplants: a predictable effect of waning herd immunity', *Lancet* 2003; 362: 832.

31 A working group created under the auspices of the UK's Academy of Medical Sciences came to largely the same conclusion in March 2001. Led by Professor Peter Lachmann, and comprising twelve of the country's leading vaccine experts (including Professor Arie Zuckerman, who presided over the original Wakefield research at the Royal Free), the Academy noted that:

> With the record linkage possibilities in the UK, we are in a strong position to set up routine and systematic monitoring systems to detect and to assess both short and long-term adverse effects of vaccines. This would seem to be an important priority, not least to enable a rapid and informed response to allegations of vaccine-associated adverse effects

that are bound to recur and that have detrimental effects on vaccine uptake even when they have little substance.

32 See Kathleen R. Stratton and colleagues, 'Adverse events associated with childhood vaccines other than pertussis and rubella', *JAMA* 1994; 271: 1602–5. The UK's Department of Health argues vigorously that all the measures proposed in this Institute of Medicine committee report are already in place. But it is far from clear that this is so. There is no effective mechanism at present to study vaccine safety before vaccines are made widely available. This is an inevitable failing of clinical trials, rather than a specific failing of vaccine evaluation. And if the means to be sure of safety after a vaccine has been licensed were in place, one wonders why the Department has not done more to reassure the public. To be fair, in my conversations with Department of Health officials it is clear that they firmly believe – in genuinely good faith – that the measures they have implemented to protect the public from unwanted effects caused by and unnecessary scares associated with vaccines are robust and effective. Yet the same officials also concede that they have been slow to make their case, disclose information, and show that they have not only listened to public concern but also responded to those concerns. However one cuts this issue, there has been a substantial failure at the heart of government. The Department of Health might argue that this failure is one of communication only. It is my contention that this failure goes further.

CHAPTER 2: SCIENCE FRICTION

1 See Stuart Hampshire, *Justice is Conflict*, Princeton University Press, 2000. Hampshire's argument was first made in his presidential address given at the American Philosophical Association on 29 March 1991. His lecture was then entitled, 'Justice is Strife'. Hampshire died on 13 June 2004, aged eighty-nine.

2 This present book is, in one sense, a reply to Hampshire concerning a very specific part of the public sphere of human conversation – namely, science in society. Certainly, it is his writing that has driven many of the ideas set out here.

3 See 'This orchestrated campaign must not be allowed to stifle real

debate on MMR', *Independent*, 24 February 2004, 16. John Reid, the Secretary of State for Health, shot back the following day with a denial. He called the newspaper's claim of an orchestrated campaign 'unfounded and misleading'.

4 Which several MPs successfully found. See, for example, Mark Henderson, 'MMR doctors challenged over child spinal taps', *The Times*, 26 February 2004, 1.

5 See Sam Coates, 'MPs call for full retraction of study linking MMR to autism', *The Times*, 5 March 2004, 6.

6 Letter dated 9 March 2004, from the Second Clerk of the Committee, Emily Commander.

7 This we did. The final report of the UK Parliamentary Science and Technology Committee's inquiry into scientific publications was published in July 2004. It made no mention of the MMR vaccine.

8 See J. W. Lee and colleagues, 'Autism, inflammatory bowel disease, and MMR vaccine', *Lancet* 1998; 351: 905–9.

9 See, for example, D. R. Walker, 'Autism, inflammatory bowel disease, and MMR vaccine', *Lancet* 1998; 351: 1355–8.

10 See Robert T. Chen and Frank DeStefano, 'Vaccine safety', *Lancet* 1998; 352: 63–4.

11 See Frank DeStefano and Robert T. Chen, 'Negative association between MMR and autism', *Lancet* 1999; 353: 1987–8.

12 See M. A. Afzal and colleagues, 'Clinical safety issues of measles, mumps, and rubella vaccines', *Bulletin of the World Health Organization* 2000; 78: 199–204.

13 See Elizabeth Miller, 'Commentary', *Archives of Disease in Childhood* 2001; 85: 273–4; 'MMR vaccine: review of benefits and risks', *Journal of Infection* 2002; 44: 1–6; and 'Measles–mumps–rubella vaccine and the development of autism', *Seminars in Pediatric Infectious Diseases* 2003; 14: 199–206.

14 See 'Interesting conflicts . . .', *Private Eye*, March 2004.

15 See David Salisbury and Joanne Yarwood, 'Public perception of immunization', *Lancet* 2004; 363: 1324.

16 Other groups of scientists also exist to advise government. One, for example, is the Council for Science and Technology. This forum of élite scientists was created in 1993 to provide a direct line of scientific advice to the Prime Minister. Ian Gibson, the chairman of the

Parliamentary Science and Technology Committee, has called the council 'just another talking shop'. Reconstituted in March 2004, it includes the director of the Wellcome Trust (Mark Walport), the President of the Academy of Medical Sciences (Keith Peters), the Government's chief scientific adviser (David King), and a Nobel Prize winner (Paul Nurse). The kindest comment that one can offer is that its influence on government is so hard to discern that it must be very great indeed.

17 See Kenneth C. Calman, 'Communication of risk: choice, consent, and trust', *Lancet* 2002; 360: 166–8.

18 See, for example, Paul A. Offit and Susan E. Coffin, 'Communicating science to the public: MMR vaccine and autism', *Vaccine* 2003; 22: 1–6. These American authors wrote: '. . . news reports about MMR vaccine and autism have been more interesting than informative – reports often include emotional and dramatic stories of parents concerned that their children were harmed by MMR vaccine rather than details of specific scientific studies.' A similar conclusion was reached by a group of UK media commentators, who found that: 'Although almost all scientific experts rejected the claim of a link between MMR and autism, 53% of those surveyed at the height of the media coverage of the issues assumed that because both sides of the debate received equal media coverage, there must be equal evidence for each. Only 23% of the population were aware that the bulk of evidence favoured supporters of the vaccine.' See 'Towards a Better Map: Science, the Public, and the Media', Economic and Social Research Council, 2003.

19 See Maggie Evans and colleagues, 'Parents' perspectives on the MMR immunization: a focus group study', *British Journal of General Practice* 2001; 51: 904–10; Karen A. Roberts and colleagues, 'Factors affecting uptake of childhood immunizations', *Lancet* 2002; 360: 1596–9; M. Petrovic and colleagues, 'Parents' attitude towards the second dose of measles, mumps, and rubella vaccine', *Communicable Disease and Public Health* 2003; 6: 325–9.

20 See Public Health Sciences Working Group, 'Public Health Sciences: challenges and opportunities', Wellcome Trust, 2004.

21 See 'Dissent must be aired', *Times Higher Education Supplement*, 27 February 2004, 4.

22 See John Walker-Smith, 'Autism, bowel inflammation and measles', *Lancet* 2002; 359: 705–6; Simon Murch, 'Separating inflammation from speculation in autism', *Lancet* 2003; 362: 1498–9; and Peter Harvey, 'MMR and autism: the debate continues', *Lancet* 2004; 363: 568.

23 See Ann and Martin Hewitt and ten other parents, 'MMR campaign must not hinder research', *Daily Telegraph*, 22 March 2004, 23; and Nina Goswami and Jon Ungoed-Thomas, 'Human cost of MMR scare', *Sunday Times*, 4 April 2004, 1. The poisonous conflict over Wakefield's work continued months after the *Lancet*'s imbroglio. Brian Deer continued his investigations for the *Sunday Times*, identifying further possible discrepancies in a research paper published in *Molecular Pathology* concerning the origin of measles genetic material in tissue samples from children with autism. See 'New doubts cast on MMR study data', *Sunday Times*, 25 April, 11.

CHAPTER 3: THE DAWN OF MCSCIENCE

Acknowledgement: Parts of this chapter first appeared as a review-essay published in the *New York Review of Books*, 'The dawn of McScience', 11 March 2004, 7–9.

1 See Andreas Whittam Smith, 'MMR, Conrad Black, and the dilemma of reconciling conflicting interests', *Independent*, 23 February 2004, 31.

2 See George Monbiot, 'The corporate stooges who nobble serious science', *Guardian*, 24 February 2004, 26; and 'Starved of the truth', *Guardian*, 9 March 2004, 23.

3 See 'All above board', *New Scientist*, 6 March 2004, 3.

4 See 'In no one's best interest', *Nature*, 4 March 2004, 1.

5 See Kenneth J. Rothman, 'Conflict of interest: The new McCarthyism in science', *JAMA* 1993; 269: 2782–4.

6 See Tim Utton, 'A conflict of interest over MMR? Now look how 19 Government experts are connected', *Daily Mail*, 25 February 2004, 10.

7 See 'Misled over MMR', *Observer*, 22 February 2004, 28. An editorialist wrote that, 'The *Lancet* must introduce a rigorous and transparent process for establishing conflicts of interest.'

8 See Frank Davidoff and colleagues, 'Sponsorship, authorship, and accountability', *Lancet* 2001; 358: 854–6; Astrid James and Richard Horton, '*The Lancet*'s policy on conflicts of interest', *Lancet* 2003; 361: 8–9; and Astrid James and colleagues, '*The Lancet*'s policy on conflicts of interest – 2004', *Lancet* 2004; 363: 2–3.

9 See S. Y. H. Kim and colleagues, 'Potential research participants' views regarding researcher and institutional financial conflicts of interest', *Journal of Medical Ethics* 2004; 30: 73–9.

10 Rowman and Littlefield, 2003.

11 See Justin E. Bekelman et al., 'Scope and impact of financial conflicts of interest in biomedical research', *JAMA*, 22 January 2003, 454–65.

12 The NIH is currently embroiled in controversy following allegations, first reported in the *Los Angeles Times* on 7 December 2003, that money received by some of the agency's top scientists has biased research decisions. NIH director Elias Zerhouni responded quickly by setting up committees to investigate these 'important' claims.

13 See Bertrand Russell, 'General effects of scientific technique', *The Impact of Science on Society*, Routledge, 1985, 29–54.

14 See Robert K. Merton, 'Science and the social order', *Philosophy of Science*, Vol. 5 (1938), 321–37.

15 See Steven Shapin, *A Social History of Truth*, University of Chicago Press, 1995.

16 See Sidney Taurel, 'Hands off my industry', *Wall Street Journal*, 3 November 2003, A14.

17 See William F. Raub, 'The emerging partnerships among the National Institutes of Health, Academic Health Centers, and industry', *Preparing for Science in the 21st Century*, Association of Academic Health Centers, 1991.

18 See Eric G. Campbell et al., 'Data withholding in academic genetics', *JAMA*, 23 January 2002, 473–80.

19 See Kevin A. Schulman et al., 'A national survey of provisions in clinical-trial agreements between medical schools and industry sponsors', *New England Journal of Medicine*, 24 October 2002, 1335–41.

20 See Jon Thompson, Patricia Baird and Jocelyn Downie, *The Olivieri Report*, James Lorimer, 2001.

21 See Derek Bok, *Universities in the Marketplace*, Princeton University

Press, 2003, and Daniel Callahan, *What Price Better Health*, University of California Press, 2003.

22 Few physicians are prepared to discuss openly their links with industry. A rare exception was recently provided by a UK professor of medicine, Edwin Gale. See his 'Between two cultures: The expert-clinician and the pharmaceutical industry', *Clinical Medicine*, November/December 2003, 538–41.

23 Although a variable but often considerable proportion of the 'scientific' content is promotional too – typically in the guise of sponsored satellite meetings at which speakers, in exchange for substantial fees, will lecture to a specially invited audience with a particular product in mind.

24 One study done in Scotland, for example, found that the pharmaceutical industry paid for about half of the meetings attended by doctors. See Philip Rutledge and colleagues, 'Do doctors rely on pharmaceutical industry funding to attend conferences and do they perceive that this creates a bias in their drug selection? Results from a questionnaire survey', *Pharmacoepidemiology and Drug Safety* 2003; 12: 663–7.

25 See H. T. Stelfox et al., 'Conflict of interest in the debate over calcium-channel antagonists', *New England Journal of Medicine*, 8 January 1998, 101–6.

26 See, for example, Antony Barnett, 'Revealed: How drug firms "hoodwink" medical journals', *Observer*, 7 December 2003; and Alexander C. Tsai, 'Conflicts between commercial and scientific interests in pharmaceutical advertising for medical journals', *International Journal of Health Services* 2003; 33: 751–68. In one recent report, scientists who were responsible for conducting clinical trials into the safety of antidepressants for children and adolescents were accused of exaggerating the benefits and downplaying the harm of these drugs. The scientists who were studying the scientists questioned the degree of critical scrutiny provided by the journals that published these trials. They wrote of their concern 'that biased reporting and overconfident recommendations in treatment guidelines may mislead doctors, patients, and families'. See Jon N. Jureidini and colleagues, 'Efficacy and safety of antidepressants for children and adolescents', *BMJ* 2004; 328: 879–83.

27 See Lisa A. Bero et al., 'The publication of sponsored symposiums in medical journals', *New England Journal of Medicine*, 15 October 1992, 1135–40; and Paula A. Rochon et al., 'Evaluating the quality of articles published in journal supplements compared with the quality of those published in the parent journal', *JAMA*, 13 July, 1994, 108–13.

28 See An-Wen Chan and colleagues, 'Empirical evidence for selective reporting of outcomes in randomized trials', *JAMA* 2004; 291: 2457–65.

29 See Craig J. Whittington and colleagues, 'Selective serotonin reuptake inhibitors in childhood depression: systematic review of published versus unpublished data', *Lancet* 2004; 363: 1341–5.

30 See Arnold S. Relman and Marcia Angell, 'America's other drug problem', *New Republic*, 16 December 2002, 27–41.

31 See John Ziman, 'Non-instrumental roles of science', *Science and Engineering Ethics*, Vol. 9 (2003), 17–27.

32 In 2004, David King published a report arguing that the UK was second only to the US in the strength of its science base. He praised the UK's 'resourcefulness' in approaching industry for research funding. He wrote that, 'the United Kingdom's business investment in public research, as a proportion of public research R and D, is the highest in the world.' This seemed to him to be a cause for satisfaction. See 'The Scientific Impact of Nations', *Nature* 2004; 430: 311–16. In July, 2004, the UK government committed itself to an average annual growth in the science budget of 5.6 per cent until 2008. This increase, well above both inflation and the average annual growth of the economy, will take the proportion of national income spent on science from 1.9 per cent today to 2.5 per cent by 2014. The government argued that, 'the major challenge for the UK science base in the coming decade is to translate investment effectively into economic and public service impact, through stronger synergies with other investment from a range of public and private sources, and increased engagement with business'. There was no analysis of the potential adverse consequences of this strategy.

33 See Michael Farthing and colleagues, 'UK's failure to act on research misconduct', *Lancet* 2000; 356: 2030.

34 See Magne Nylenna and colleagues, 'Handling of scientific dishonesty in the Nordic countries', *Lancet* 1999; 354: 57–61.

CHAPTER 4: ALONE WITH AUTISM

1 Experts on autism dispute this claim. They say that the prevalence of bowel symptoms in children with autism is extremely small, perhaps no different from the rest of the (non-autistic) population. Writing in the *Sunday Times* on 11 April 2004, Wakefield wrote, 'My first duty is to my patients and I have urged and will continue to urge parents to immunize their children against the respective [measles, mumps, and rubella] diseases. If, as appears to be the case, the public simply do not trust the safety of MMR then the time has come for the authorities to reinstate parents' rights to choose the single vaccines which have been used for many years.'

2 Some newspapers described the treatment of these parents as a 'betrayal', especially when they were denied legal aid to continue their 'battle'. See, for example, David Hughes and Jenny Hope, 'MMR: The betrayal of these tragic parents', *Daily Mail*, 24 February 2004, 1; Celia Hall, 'Parents of autistic children battle on', *Daily Telegraph*, 23 February 2004, 4; and Jenny Hope, 'The fight goes on, vow MMR parents after £10 m setback', *Daily Mail*, 28 February 2004, 41. Michael Fitzpatrick, a doctor whose own son has autism, argues that the anti-vaccine campaign pursued by some parents of children with autism has 'nurtured self pity, expressed in an enduring rage against the drug companies, the medical establishment, indeed anybody who defends the vaccine'. While Fitzpatrick speaks with an authority that I could never claim – I have no direct experience of living with a child who has autism – I think his generalized adverse characterization of parents seeking a cause for their child's illness is profoundly unfortunate. To label these parents as displaying 'self-pity' was a graceless and gratuitous comment. See Michael Fitzpatrick, 'George and Sam', *BMJ* 2004; 328: 1571.

3 Wakefield, *Sunday Times*, 11 April 2004.

4 See Marlene Targ Brill, *Keys to Parenting the Child with Autism*, Barron's, 2001; Shirley Cohen, *Targeting Autism: What We Know, Don't Know, and Can Do to Help Young Children with Autism and Related Disorders*, University of California Press, 2002; Stephen B. Edelson, *Conquering Autism: Reclaiming Your Child Through Natural Therapies*, Twin Streams, 2004; Uta Frith, *Autism: Explaining the Enigma*, Blackwell, 2003; Lynn M. Hamilton, *Facing Autism: Giving Parents Reasons for Hope and Guidance for Help*, Waterbook Press,

2000; Stephanie Marohn, *The Natural Medicine Guide to Autism*, Hampton Roads, 2002; Fiona Marshall, *Living with Autism*, Sheldon Press, 2004; Chantal Sicile-Kira, *Autism Spectrum Disorders: The Complete Guide*, Vermilion, 2003; Bryna Siegel, *Helping Children with Autism Learn: Treatment Approaches for Parents and Professionals*, Oxford University Press, 2003; Patricia Stacey, *The Boy Who Loved Windows*, DaCapo Press, 2003; Adelle Jameson Tilton, *The Everything Parent's Guide to Children with Autism*, Adams Media, 2004; Diane Yapko, *Understanding Autism Spectrum Disorders*, Jessica Kingsley, 2003; and Lorna Wing, *The Autistic Spectrum: A Parents Guide to Understanding and Helping Your Child*, Ulysses Press, 2001.

5 The quotations are: 'One thing that keeps coming back time after time . . . is the central role of the gut in this disorder' (Chapter 7); and 'What I am intrigued by is how this is a parent led phenomenon. [Almost] everything I've learned about this disease has come from parents' (Chapter 9).

6 See Leo Kanner, 'Autistic disturbances of affective contact', *Nervous Child* 1943; 2: 217–50.

7 See Bruno Bettelheim, 'Joey: A "mechanical" boy', *Scientific American*, March 1959, 117–27.

8 See Bernard Rimland, 'Introduction', In *Children with Autism*, edited by Michael D. Powers, Woodbine House, 2000, xix –xxvii. Rimland also has decidedly pointed views on vaccines. In 1995, he wrote in the most alarmist terms that pertussis (whooping cough) vaccination may be a cause of 'minimal brain damage . . . [and] allergy-caused encephalitis (brain inflammation), which may in turn cause autism and other brain disorders'. In 1998 he extended his thesis beyond pertussis to the MMR vaccine. He called Wakefield 'courageous' and criticized those who defended vaccines: 'The fact is, vaccines are not nearly as safe, nor anywhere near as effective, as vaccination proponents claim . . . there is an enormous amount of credible evidence that vaccines can and do cause harm . . . (the medical establishment's ferocious defence of vaccines as irrefutably safe and beneficial somehow reminds me of the *Titanic*).' See 'Children's shots: no longer a simple decision', *Autism Research Review International* 1995; 9 (1): 1; and 'Vaccinations: The overlooked factors', *Autism Research Review International* 1998; 12 (1): 1.

9 See Fred R. Volkmar and David Pauls, 'Autism', *Lancet* 2003; 362: 1133–41; Fred R. Volkmar and colleagues, 'Autism and pervasive developmental disorders', *Journal of Child Psychology and Psychiatry* 2004; 45: 135–70; Patrick F. Bolton and Paul D. Griffiths, 'Association of tuberous sclerosis of temporal lobes with autism and atypical autism', *Lancet* 1997; 349: 392–5; Patrick F. Bolton and colleagues, 'Association between idiopathic infantile macrocephaly and autism spectrum disorders', *Lancet* 2001; 358: 726–7; and Gregory L. Wallace and Darold A. Treffert, 'Head size and autism', *Lancet* 2004; 363: 1003–4.

10 See Nigel Hawkes, *The Times*, 1 April 2004, 12; and Nicolas Ramoz and colleagues, 'Linkage and association of the mitochondrial aspartate/glutamate carrier SLC25A12 gene with autism', *American Journal of Psychiatry* 2004; 161: 662–9. See also, Nigel Hawkes, 'Families chip in to find DNA that causes autism', *The Times*, 19 July 2004, 21.

11 See G. Baird and colleagues, 'Screening and surveillance for autism and pervasive developmental disorders', *Archives of Disease of Childhood* 2001; 84: 468–75.

12 See Fred R. Volkmar and Donald J. Cohen, 'Disintegrative disorders or "late-onset" autism', *Journal of Child Psychology and Psychiatry* 1989; 30: 717–24. It makes little sense to argue that the MMR vaccine is the cause of the syndrome described by Volkmar and Cohen. This late-onset condition was evident long before the MMR vaccine was ever introduced, and its prevalence has remained unchanged despite the widespread use of the triple vaccine. See, for example, Catherine Lord and colleagues, 'Regression and word loss in autistic spectrum disorders', *Journal of Child Psychology and Psychiatry* 2004; 45: 936–55.

13 See Stella Chess and colleagues, 'Behavioural consequences of congenital rubella', *Journal of Pediatrics* 1978; 93: 699–703.

14 See Michael C. Stevens and colleagues, 'Season of birth effects in autism', *Journal of Clinical and Experimental Neuropsychology* 2000; 22: 399–407.

15 See Steven Pinker, *The Blank Slate*, Penguin, 2002, 62.

16 See Simon Baron-Cohen and colleagues, 'Does the autistic child have a "theory of mind"?', *Cognition* 1985; 21: 37–46.

17 See Simon Baron-Cohen, 'The autistic child's theory of mind: A case

of specific developmental delay', *Journal of Child Psychology and Psychiatry* 1989; 30: 285–97.

18 See Simon Baron-Cohen, 'The development of a theory of mind in autism: Deviance and delay?', *Psychiatric Clinics of North America* 1991; 14: 33–51.

19 See Simon Baron-Cohen and colleagues, 'Recognition of mental state terms: Clinical findings in children with autism and a functional neuroimaging study of normal adults', *British Journal of Psychiatry* 1994; 165: 640–49; and Valerie E. Stone and colleagues, 'Frontal lobe contributions to theory of mind', *Journal of Cognitive Neuroscience* 1998; 10: 640–56.

20 See Simon Baron-Cohen, *Mindblindness*, MIT Press, 1995. For an up-to-date review of mindblindness in the context of other theories of autism see, Simon Baron-Cohen, 'The cognitive neuroscience of autism', *Journal of Neurology, Neurosurgery and Psychiatry* 2004; 75: 945–8.

21 See Simon Baron-Cohen, *The Essential Difference*, Allen Lane, 2003.

22 See Lorna Wing, 'The autistic spectrum', *Lancet* 1997; 350: 1761–6.

23 See Fiona J. Scott and colleagues, 'Prevalence of autism spectrum conditions in children aged 5–11 years in Cambridgeshire, UK', *Autism* 2002; 6: 231–7; Lorna Wing and David Potter, 'The epidemiology of autism spectrum disorders: Is the prevalence rising?', *Mental Retardation and Developmental Disabilities Research Reviews* 2002; 8: 151–61; Hershel Jick and James A. Kaye, 'Epidemiology and possible causes of autism', *Pharmacotherapy* 2003; 23: 1524–30; and Hershel Jick and James A. Kaye, 'Changes in risk of autism in the UK for birth cohorts 1990–1998', *Epidemiology* 2003; 14: 630–32. In my discussions of this problem with autism experts, Lorna Wing has identified an additional possible explanation for the rising incidence of autism. The early feeding problems that are experienced by some children with autism could have contributed to their higher infant mortality. With better child care, infant mortality rates have fallen, perhaps enabling children with autism to survive, expanding their numbers in the wider population and so giving the (false) impression of an increasing frequency of the disorder. Concerning her proposal to conduct a cohort study into the proposed link between the MMR

vaccine and autism, Wing now believes that it could only be justified if vaccination rates suffered a dramatic decline. With limited resources, priority setting for research becomes all important. Research into the MMR vaccine might take money away from other more promising areas of investigation.

24 For example, a survey of general practitioners by the National Autistic Society, completed in November 2002, found that over 40 per cent had insufficient information to make an assessment of a patient who they suspected might have autism. Forty per cent were also unaware of where to turn for support and more information. And one in ten doctors did not know how and where to refer on a child with a suspected diagnosis of autism. Given that treatment options for autism are rapidly progressing, these flaws in diagnostic and care services are profoundly troubling. See Eric Hollander and colleagues, 'Targeted treatments for symptom domains in child and adolescent autism', *Lancet* 2003; 362: 732–4.

25 This report, entitled *The Impact of Autism*, can be found on the website of the National Autistic Society (www.nas.org).

26 In 2002, the UK Government pledged a further £2.5 million for autism research. The funds went to the Medical Research Council in order to advance the research agenda set out in its 2001 report. The MRC was already spending some £1.3 million on research into autism each year. Existing studies included investigations of chromosome 15 concerning the development of autistic spectrum disorders; research into the brain pathology of autism; and the identification of psychological differences among children with autism. An MRC Steering Group, chaired by Professor Carol Dezateux and including two lay members among a team of six advisers, was established to guide implementation of the new MRC strategy. The first research grants were awarded in 2004. Several projects were funded. The largest was a study of environmental risks, including the MMR vaccine, led by Professor Jean Golding at the University of Bristol. Other new research will encompass brain injury, language and communication, and cognition.

27 Wing and Potter, 'The epidemiology of autism spectrum disorders'. See note 23 above.

28 11 May 2004.

CHAPTER 5: CAN MEASLES BE ERADICATED?

1 See Trevor Duke and Charles S. Mgone, 'Measles: not just another viral exanthem', *Lancet* 2003; 361: 763–73. There is considerable disagreement among experts about the numbers of measles infections and deaths occurring each year. The official statistics from WHO are that, in 2002, there were 760,000 deaths in the world from measles, which broke down region by region as follows:

Africa	439,000
South East Asia	198,000
Eastern Mediterranean	84,000
Western Pacific	32,000
Europe	7,000
The Americas	0
TOTAL	760,000

However, in 2004, as a result of better information about vaccination campaigns and case fatalities, WHO revised these estimates downwards to a global figure of 610,000 deaths. Another respected group of investigators has estimated the number of measles deaths in 2000 to be 103,000, a remarkably low figure when set against even the revised WHO estimate. What these wildly different numbers tell us is that the world has very poor systems for reliably estimating how many people die of particular diseases. If WHO should be able to do anything at all, it should surely be able to do this. See Gareth Jones and colleagues, 'How many child deaths can we prevent this year?', *Lancet* 2003; 362: 65–71.

2 See Peter J. Hotez and colleagues, 'Combating tropical infectious diseases: Report of the disease control priorities in developing countries project', *Clinical Infectious Diseases* 2004; 38: 1–8.

3 See Heikki Peltola and colleagues, 'No measles in Finland', *Lancet* 1997; 350: 1364–5.

4 See Mark A. Miller and colleagues, 'A model to estimate the potential economic benefits of measles eradication for the United States', *Vaccine* 1998; 16: 1917–22; and Helene Carabin and W. John Edmunds, 'Future savings from measles eradication in industrialized

countries', *Journal of Infectious Diseases* 2003; 187 (Suppl 1): 529–35.

5 See *Strategic Plan for Measles and Congenital Rubella Infection in the European Region of WHO*, 2003.

6 See 'Measles eradication: Recommendations from a meeting cosponsored by the WHO, the PAHO, and CDC', *MMWR* 1997; 46: 1–20. Measles, like polio and smallpox, is theoretically eradicable. The criteria for eradication are: first, that human beings are the only reservoir able to maintain the existence of the virus; second, that there are good diagnostic tests for measles available; and, third, that there is a need for only one type of vaccine (because there is only type of virus). Measles fulfils all three criteria. The most impressive campaign of measles elimination has undoubtedly been that organized by the Pan American Health Organization. Its three-tiered immunization policy has largely erased the measles virus from the human population of the Americas. See Bradley S. Hersh and colleagues, 'Review of regional measles surveillance data in the Americas, 1996–99', *Lancet* 2000; 355: 1943–8.

7 See *Measles Reduction and Regional Elimination Strategic Plan 2001–2005*, Geneva, WHO, 2001.

8 See *Weekly Epidemiological Record* 2004; 3: 13–24.

9 See Robin Biellik and colleagues, 'First 5 years of measles elimination in Southern Africa: 1996–2000', *Lancet* 2002; 359: 1564–8.

10 See R. L. de Swart and colleagues, 'Measles in a Dutch hospital introduced by an immuno-compromised infant from Indonesia infected with a new virus genotype', *Lancet* 2000; 355: 201–2.

11 See N. S. Wairagkar and colleagues, 'Acute renal failure with neurological involvement in adults associated with measles virus isolation', *Lancet* 1999; 354: 992–5; and Hilton C. Whittle and colleagues, 'Effect of subclinical infection on maintaining immunity against measles in vaccinated children in West Africa', *Lancet* 1999; 353: 98–101.

12 See Teresa Michele Marshall and colleagues, 'Nosocomial outbreaks – a potential threat to the elimination of measles?' *Journal of Infectious Diseases* 2003; 187 (Suppl. 1): 597–601.

13 See C. Kamugisha and colleagues, 'An outbreak of measles in Tanzanian refugee camps', *Journal of Infectious Diseases* 2003; 187 (Suppl. 1): 558–62.

14 See Rory Carroll, 'Polio strikes in Botswana as virus races across Africa', *Guardian*, 16 April 2004, 15; *Weekly Epidemiological Record* 2004; 79: 121–5; Jeevan Vasagar, 'Polio jabs a US plot, claim Nigerian Muslims', *Guardian*, 25 February 2004, 16; and Sarah Boseley, 'Polio outbreak threatens Africa', *Guardian*, 23 June 2004, 14. The polio vaccine has also been the subject of safety concerns. Some of the earliest doses of the polio vaccine used in the 1960s were contaminated with a virus called SV40. This virus is known to cause cancer in laboratory animals. There is understandable concern, although no absolute proof, that it might do the same in man. See Debbie Bookchin, 'Vaccine scandal revives cancer fear', *New Scientist* 10 July 2004, 6–7.

15 These arguments are reviewed in greater detail by Felicity T. Cutts and R. Steinglass, 'Should measles be eradicated?', *BMJ* 1998; 316: 765–7; Mohamed Ibrahim Ali Omar, 'Measles: A disease that has to be eradicated', *Annals of Tropical Paediatrics* 1999; 19: 125–34; Walter A. Orenstein and colleagues, 'Measles eradication: Is it in our future?', *American Journal of Public Health* 2000; 90: 1521–5; Sheila Davey, 'Measles eradication still a long way off', *Bulletin of the World Health Organization* 2001; 79: 584–5; Isao Arita and colleagues, 'Eradication of infectious diseases', *Japanese Journal of Infectious Diseases* 2004; 57: 1–6; Oliver W. C. Morgan, 'Following in the footsteps of smallpox: Can we achieve the global eradication of measles?', *BMC International Health and Human Rights* 2004; 4: 1; and Ciro A. de Quadros, 'Can measles be eradicated globally?', *Bulletin of the World Health Organization* 2004; 82: 134–8.

16 See Athmanunah Dilraj and colleagues, 'Response to different measles vaccine strains given by aerosol and subcutaneous routes to schoolchildren', *Lancet* 2000; 355: 798–803.

17 See N. S. Wairagkar and colleagues, 'Isolation of measles virus below 4 months of age during an outbreak in Pune, India', *Lancet* 1998; 351: 495–6. There is a contrary view emerging about the need to vaccinate at younger ages. The key to protecting children younger than the age for measles vaccination might be to ensure that measles virus does not circulate among other members of the family and community. Interrupting virus circulation in older children – the main source of measles for infants – may be a better strategy for protecting young

children than vaccination. This same optimism extends to the control of measles in the crowded cities of developing nations. The current measles vaccine, assuming high enough coverage rates, according to sources within the World Health Organization, could control measles in these difficult settings. As one measles expert put it to me, 'After forty years we have finally learned how to properly use this vaccine.'

18 See Mike M. Putz and colleagues, 'Experimental vaccines against measles in a world of changing epidemiology', *International Journal for Parasitology* 2003; 33: 525–45; Gregory J. Atkins and S. Louise Cosby, 'Is an improved measles–mumps–rubella vaccine necessary or feasible?', *Critical Reviews in Immunology* 2003; 23: 323–38; Diane E. Webster and colleagues, 'Successful boosting of a DNA measles immunization with an oral plant-derived measles virus vaccine', *Journal of Virology* 2002; 76: 7910–12, and Sallie R. Permar and colleagues, 'Role of CD8+ lymphocytes in control and clearance of measles virus infection of Rhesus monkeys', *Journal of Virology* 2003; 77: 4396–400.

19 See Mary-Lill Garly and Peter Aaby, 'The challenge of improving the efficacy of measles vaccine', *Acta Tropica* 2003; 85: 1–17. There is another reason why it may be wise – perhaps even impossible – to end measles vaccination programmes. Stopping immunization completely would introduce the risk that other measles-like viruses, which presently circulate in animal populations, could jump species and cause significant harm to human beings. It seems there is a growing consensus that measles vaccination is forever. See Koert J. Stittelaar and colleagues, 'Vaccination against measles: a neverending story', *Expert Reviews in Vaccines* 2002; 1: 151–9.

20 See Richard Horton, 'Bioterrorism: The extreme politics of public health', In *Global Public Health: A New Era*, edited by Robert Beaglehole, Oxford University Press, 2003, 209–25.

21 See Peter Strebel and colleagues, 'The unfinished measles immunization agenda', *Journal of Infectious Diseases* 2003; 187 (Suppl. 1): 51–7.

22 See the collection of five articles published in *Lancet* in June and July 2003 – in particular, Robert E. Black and colleagues, 'Where and why are 10 million children dying every year?', *Lancet* 2003; 361: 2226–34; Gareth Jones and colleagues, 'How many child deaths can

we prevent this year?', *Lancet* 2003; 362: 65–71; and Jennifer Bryce and colleagues, 'Reducing child mortality: Can public health deliver?', *Lancet* 2003; 362: 159–64.

CHAPTER 6: THE MANUFACTURE OF FEAR

1 Arnold, 2004.

2 See David A. Grimes and Kenneth F. Schulz, 'An overview of clinical research: The lay of the land', *Lancet* 2002; 359: 57–61.

3 See James E. Enstrom and Geoffrey C. Kabat, 'Environmental tobacco smoke and tobacco related mortality in a prospective study of Californians, 1960–98', *BMJ* 2003; 326: 1057–61.

4 Interestingly, the dispute about this *BMJ* paper also centred around alleged conflicts of interest. In 1996, Enstrom wrote to Max Eisenberg, director of the Center for Indoor Air Pollution, an organization largely funded by the tobacco industry, boasting that he had 'done consulting and research on passive smoking' on behalf of tobacco companies R. J. Reynolds and Philip Morris. He claimed that his results contradicted received wisdom about the risks of environmental tobacco smoke. And he sought further funding for work that he assured Eisenberg would 'yield important new findings on the health effects of passive smoking'.

5 See Richard Horton, 'ICRF: From mayhem to meltdown', *Lancet* 1997; 350: 1043–4.

6 See Peter C. Gøtzsche and Ole Olsen, 'Is screening for breast cancer with mammography justifiable?' *Lancet* 2000; 355: 129–34; and Ole Olsen and Peter C. Gøtzsche, 'Cochrane review on screening for breast cancer with mammography', *Lancet* 2001; 358: 1340–2.

7 See Robert May, 'GM warriors have killed the debate', *Guardian*, 25 November 2003, 24.

8 The committee also described a third category of science writing – namely, the specialist scientific press, written by scientists for scientists. They dismissed this group, which includes medical journals such as the *Lancet*. This seems mistaken to me, since, although we are not read by the public very often, we are read by journalists and so influence news agendas and the broad brush of public conversation.

9 It is worth noting, however, that these events often cater to the converted – that is, to those already interested in science. In an important

report published in October 2000, entitled *Science and the Public* and commissioned jointly by the UK's Office of Science and Technology and the Wellcome Trust, a variety of (sometimes contradictory) public attitudes to science was revealed. While 80 per cent of those surveyed recognized the value of science to society, almost a fifth believed that the benefits of science did not outweigh its harm. Four out of ten people believed that science was advancing so fast that it could not be properly controlled by government.

10 See Geoff Mulgan, 'The media's lies poison our system', *Guardian*, 7 May 2004, 24.

11 See Eva Benelli, 'The role of the media in steering public opinion on healthcare issues', *Health Policy* 2003; 63: 179–86.

12 See Tim Radford, 'Influence and power of the media', *Lancet* 1996; 347: 1533–5.

13 See Cass R. Sunstein, *Risk and Reason*, Cambridge University Press, 2002.

14 See, for example, Richard Keeble, *Ethics for Journalists*, Routledge, 2001; Ian Hargreaves, *Journalism: Truth or Dare*, Oxford University Press, 2003; and Jack Fuller, *News Values*, University of Chicago Press, 1996.

15 See Victor Cohn, 'A perspective from the press: How to help reporters tell the truth (sometimes)', *Statistics in Medicine* 2001; 20: 1341–6. Cohn died in February 2000. One of my most prized possessions is a personally signed copy of his book.

16 There are oblique signs that British journalism is entering a new era marked by values emphasizing precision and fairness. In the wake of the Hutton Inquiry into the death of David Kelly, the BBC has undergone a prolonged and unprecedented period of journalistic self-analysis, culminating in the Neil Report, published in June 2004. This report identified five core journalistic values: truth and accuracy, serving the public interest, impartiality and diversity of opinion, independence, and accountability. There are sceptics, however. Writing in *The Times* (25 June 2004), Simon Jenkins called the BBC's new focus on values 'drivel'. Interestingly, 'serving the public interest' does not mean protecting existing public health systems, such as vaccination programmes. Instead, this phrase means reporting 'stories of significance'. Balance means 'reflecting all significant strands of opinion'

and 'exploring the range and conflict of views'. There is nothing about balance being judged by appraising the totality of evidence for or against a particular opinion or view. The Hutton Inquiry offered an opportunity for news organizations to pause for reflection about their own roles in reporting and generating news. It is not at all clear that this opportunity has been seized.

17 See Niccolò Machiavelli, *Discourses on Livy*, Oxford University Press, 2003.

APPENDIX

1 Wakefield A.J., Murch S.H., Anthony A., et al. Ileal-lymphoid-nodular hyperplasia, non-specific colitis, and pervasive developmental disorder in children. *Lancet* 1998; 351: 637–41.

2 In 1998, the *Lancet* required that: 'The Editor needs to be informed [of any conflicts of interest] and will discuss with you [the authors] whether or not disclosure in the journal is necessary. All sources of funding must be disclosed, as an acknowledgement in the text.'

3 See http://www.publicationethics.org.uk/cope1999/gpp/dealing.phtml.

4 Two final, frustrating, and entirely avoidable examples. First, in August 2004, the UK government faced yet another communications disaster over childhood vaccines. The Department of Health had tried quietly to alert doctors to a change in routine childhood immunization programmes. But a leak provoked the *Daily Telegraph* (7 August 2004) to announce 'Sweeping changes to baby vaccines'. The newspaper reported that a new five-in-one jab was to be introduced in September 2004. This single vaccine included diphtheria, tetanus, acellular pertussis, inactivated polio and *Haemophilus influenzae* type B components.

To be sure, a combined vaccine was a substantial improvement on the old regimen. The live oral polio element was being replaced by an injectable inactivated vaccine, thereby eliminating the risk of vaccine associated paralytic polio. An acellular pertussis vaccine would cause fewer adverse reactions than the existing whole-cell vaccine. And a mercury-containing preservative, thiomersal, was being removed completely 'as a precautionary measure'. These changes should have been grounds for praise. But the government's inept disclosure of this new vaccination policy allowed the *Daily Mail* (9 August 2004) to claim, fairly, on its front page, 'Chaos over 5-in-1 baby jab'. Concerns over safety trumped good news.

The second example came in the same month. The chairman of the UK's Joint Committee on Vaccination and Immunisation (JCVI), Professor Michael Langman, was outed as receiving financial support from Merck, Sharp, and Dohme, one of the pharmaceutical companies, together with Aventis Pasteur, responsible for manufacturing the new five-in-one vaccine (Pediacel). His complete disclosure of this conflict of interest on the JCVI's website did nothing to allay public anxiety about his personal dual commitment – to the corporate funder of his academic research programme in Birmingham and to the committee responsible for advising government on vaccination policy. Here was a sensitive conflict of interest that should have been foreseen. It was not. The story of Andrew Wakefield and the MMR vaccine has a peculiar habit of repeating itself.

INDEX

Index